Case Studies in Endocrinology for the House Officer

OTHER BOOKS IN THE CASE STUDIES FOR THE HOUSE OFFICER SERIES

edited by Lawrence P. Levitt, M.D.

Hauser, Levitt, and Weiner
Case Studies in Neurology for the House Officer
1986/256 pages/36 figures/ #3899-0

Tomb and Christensen
Case Studies in Psychiatry for the House Officer
1987/about 256 pages/#8339-2

Heger
Case Studies in Cardiology for the House Officer
1987/about 250 pages/ illustrated/#3945-8

Solomon and Sisti
Case Studies in Neurosurgery for the House Officer
1987/about 250 pages/ illustrated/#7858-5

Case Studies in Endocrinology for the House Officer

Warner M. Burch, M.D.
*Departments of Medicine and Pharmacology
Duke University Medical Center
Durham, North Carolina*

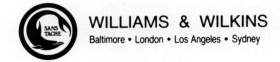

WILLIAMS & WILKINS
Baltimore • London • Los Angeles • Sydney

Editor: Kimberly Kist
Associate Editor: Linda Napora
Copy Editor: JoAnne Janowiak
Illustration Planning: Wayne Hubbel
Production: Raymond E. Reter

Copyright © 1987
Williams & Wilkins
428 East Preston Street
Baltimore, MD 21202, U.S.A.

All rights reserved. This book is protected by copyright. No part of this book may be reproduced in any form or by any means, including photocopying, or utilized by any information storage and retrieval system without written permission from the copyright owner.

Accurate indications, adverse reactions, and dosage schedules for drugs are provided in this book, but it is possible that they may change. The reader is urged to review the package information data of the manufacturers of the medications mentioned.

Printed in the United States of America

Library of Congress Cataloging in Publication Data

Burch, Warner M.
  Case studies in endocrinology for the house officer.

  (Case studies for the house officer)
  Includes bibliographies and index.
   1. Endocrine glands—Diseases—Case studies. I. Title. II. Series. [DNLM: 1. Endocrinology—case studies. WK 100 B947c]
RC649.5.B87 1987   616.4   86-18907
ISBN 0-683-01130-8

86 87 88 89 90   10 9 8 7 6 5 4 3 2 1

Series Editor's Foreword

The series, Case Studies for the House Officer, has been designed to teach medicine by a case study approach. It is considered a supplement to the parent House Officer Series which provides information in a problem-oriented format. Endocrinology for the House Officer has proved very popular with house officers and medical students. In Case Studies in Endocrinology for the House Officer, Dr. Burch has compiled an impressive series of interesting cases that cover most common endocrinologic problems. He has added thoughtful "Pearls" and "Pitfalls," and simplified diagrams of important metabolic pathways. The book should be a useful and enjoyable learning experience for students of endocrinology.

Lawrence P. Levitt, M.D.
Senior Consultant in Neurology
Lehigh Valley Hospital Center
Allentown, Pennsylvania

Clinical Associate Professor of Neurology
Hahnemann University and
Temple University School of Medicine

About the Author

Warner M. Burch, M.D., wrote the companion book for the House Officer series, Endocrinology for the House Officer. A Phi Beta Kappa graduate of Wake Forest College, he attended Bowman Gray School of Medicine as a William Neal Reynolds Scholar. After a rotating internship at Charlotte Memorial Hospital, Dr. Burch completed his medicine residency and fellowship in endocrinology at Duke University Medical Center. While in the military, he taught students in U.S. Navy and Air Force Physicians' Assistants Programs. Dr. Burch holds a Clinical Investigator Award from the National Institutes of Health and the rank of Assistant Professor of Medicine and Assistant Professor of Pharmacology. He is also Director of the Medical Endocrine Laboratory at Duke.

Preface

Case Studies in Endocrinology for the House Officer presents endocrine problems often encountered in medical practice. The author chose patients that illustrate key questions and problems in endocrinology. The format is similar to other books in the series of Case Studies for the House Officer. Some cases are easy to diagnose and manage; others offer therapeutic challenges that baffle "pat" answers. Each case has a Clue which either seals the diagnosis or points one to further studies. Pertinent laboratory data are often included [in brackets] within the Answer section of each case. The Pearls and Pitfalls sections are not inclusive. Many will think of other facets of each case that might be included in these sections. The author would appreciate any feedback and tips that might be included in future revisions. We all remain students of medicine and servants to others.

Warner M. Burch, M.D.

Acknowledgments

Writing a book requires time and support from many people. I thank my patients for the opportunity to share their problems in words and in pictures. Several of our fellows (Shawnee Weir, M.D.; Jeanne Lucas, M.D.; John Ch'ng, M.D.) and associates (Mack Harrell, M.D.; Kenneth Lyles, M.D.) offered pertinent comments and suggestions. My family continues to support my effort and deserves recognition. I love you: Vivian, Pweebe, Greta, Marcus, Joshua, and Seth.

Contents

Series Editor's Foreword	v
About the Author	vii
Preface	ix
Acknowledgments	xi

CASES

1.	Menstrual Irregularity and Facial Plethora	1
2.	Persistent Hypokalemia	12
3.	Incidental Adrenal Mass	21
4.	Spells	29
5.	Severe Weakness and Rectal Bleeding	36
6.	Weakness and Hyperpigmentation	42
7.	Anterior Neck Mass	49
8.	Nervous Patient with Abnormal Thyroid Studies	57
9.	Thyroid Nodule	62
10.	Unilateral Neck Mass	72
11.	Pruritus and Weight Loss	79
12.	Goiter and Atrial Fibrillation	86
13.	Nodular Thyroid Gland	93
14.	Elderly Woman with Decreased Hearing	100
15.	Severe Headache and Decreased Vision	108
16.	Underbite	114
17.	Milky Breast Discharge and Absent Menses	122
18.	Excessive Thirst and Polyuria	129
19.	Impotence	139
20.	Hirsutism	149

xiv CONTENTS

21.	Teenager with Amenorrhea	159
22.	Hypoglycemia	168
23.	Weakness and "Drawing" of the Hands	177
24.	Asymptomatic Hypercalcemia	186
25.	Sudden-Onset Back Pain	197
26.	Facial Swelling and Diabetes Mellitus	207
27.	Diabetes Mellitus Type II	218
28.	Diabetes and Control	226
29.	Fallen Foot Arch	236
30.	Diabetes Mellitus and Surgery	245

SHOW AND TELL (Cases 31-41) 253

INDEX 279

MENSTRUAL IRREGULARITY AND FACIAL PLETHORA

CASE 1: K.S., a 21-year-old college senior, presented because she had not had a menstrual period in 6 months. Her menses were regular until a year ago, but then became irregular for several months and finally ceased. She had noticed a 10-lb weight gain despite regular participation in an aerobics program. She was most distressed by facial fullness and fine, downy hair over her upper lip. Her mother commented that her cheeks were as "rosy as a cherubim." Her medical history was unremarkable except for the fact that she had had intermittent asthmatic attacks since age 6, but there had been no attacks in the last year.

Her weight was 129 lb; height, 64 inches; BP, 125/85; pulse, 70/min. Her face was full with ruddy cheeks. Vellus hair was present over the upper lip and sideburn area. No thoracic or abdominal striae were seen. A 3-cm area of ecchymosis over the right medial malleolus was noted. Both supraclaviclar fossa seemed full. The pelvic exam was normal; there was no uterine enlargement. The remainder of her exam was normal.

2 CASE STUDIES IN ENDOCRINOLOGY

ENDOCRINE CLUE: Photograph of lower extremity.

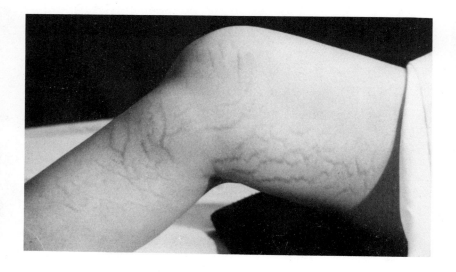

QUESTIONS:

1. What is the most likely diagnosis?

2. What studies should you order?

3. The studies you have ordered confirmed the diagnosis. What other studies would you recommend?

4. What is the treatment for this disorder?

5. What do you tell the patient about the effectiveness of therapy?

4   CASE STUDIES IN ENDOCRINOLOGY

ANSWERS:

1. The history of amenorrhea and weight gain in a 21-year-old female suggests pregnancy, but the physical exam did not confirm this.   Mild hirsutism and obesity are common in polycystic ovarian syndrome (PCOD), but the onset of menstrual abnormality is relatively late for PCOD.   The recent onset of amenorrhea, improvement in asthma, facial plethora, and the striae over the legs suggest hypercortisolism as the most likely diagnosis. The presence of striae over the calves (CLUE) in a patient with minimal weight gain should make you think of glucocorticoid excess.

2. An overnight dexamethasone study in the outpatient setting is useful to assess whether there is glucocorticoid excess. Dexamethasone 1 mg is taken between 11 PM and midnight, and a serum cortisol is drawn between 8 and 9 AM the following morning.   This level should be < 5 µg/dl. *[Her serum cortisol after taking dexamethasone at bedtime was 18 µg/dl.]* Studies to confirm hypercortisolism include a 24-hour urine for 17-hydroxycorticoids (17-OHCS) and urine free cortisol (UC). *[Urine study findings were 17-OHCS, 11 mg/gm creatinine (normal, 2.0-6.5 mg/gm Cr), and UC, 89 µg/gm creatinine (normal, < 35 µg/gm Cr).]*   These elevated levels established the diagnosis of Cushing's syndrome, but not the etiology of the hypercortisolism.   Use the diagram on the following page to orient your thoughts.

Cushing's Syndrome

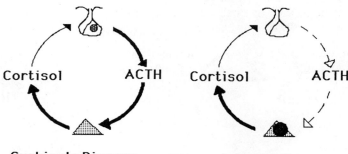

3. <u>The source of the hypercortisolism should be sought</u>. The history needs to exclude exogenous administration of glucocorticoids. Several biochemical studies have been proposed to differentiate the categories of endogenous Cushing's syndrome (<u>Cushing's disease or pituitary-dependent adrenal hyperplasia, adrenal adenoma, or ectopic adrenocorticotropic hormone [ACTH] syndrome</u>). These include Liddle's classic dexamethasone studies, single overnight high-dose dexamethasone suppression, and metyrapone loading. The author prefers the protocol using Liddle's criteria. Baseline 24-hour urine is collected for 17-OHCS and UC for two days (days 1 and 2). Dexamethasone 0.5 mg is given by mouth every 6 hours for a total of eight doses (days 3 and 4). Another 24-hour urine is collected on day 4 to determine 17-OHCS and UC. This amount of dexamethasone (low dose: 2 mg/day) suppresses the normal corticotroph, but in patients with Cushing's syndrome (any state of hypercortisolism) the 24-hour urine 17-OHCS and UC will not suppress to < 2.5 mg/gm creatinine or < 25 µg/24 hours, respectively. *[On low dose dexamethasone, this patient's urine 17-OHCS remained elevated at 9 mg/gm creatinine and*

the UC was 89 µg/24 hours on low dose dexamethasone.] In Cushing's disease the corticotrophs within the pituitary adenoma remain sensitive to glucocorticoid inhibition but only at much higher doses of dexamethasone.

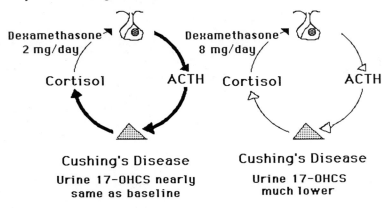

Thus, dexamethasone 2.0 mg is given by mouth every 6 hours for 8 doses (days 5 and 6) and a 24-hour urine is collected on day 6 for 17-OHCS determination. With this high dose dexamethasone (8 mg/day), patients with Cushing's disease have urine 17-OHCS < 50% of baseline values of days 1 and 2, whereas patients with hypercortisolism due to adrenal adenoma/carcinoma or ectopic ACTH syndrome have no to little suppression of the 17-OHCS. [This patient's urine 17-OHCS was 2.1 mg/gm Cr and the UC was 24 µg/24 hours on high dose dexamethasone.] The reliability of the 50% criterion for suppression in Cushing's disease is somewhat arbitrary since some patients with Cushing's disease may suppress only 35%. However, there is always significant lowering of urine 17-OHCS with high dose dexamethasone in pituitary-dependent adrenal hyperplasia.

MENSTRUAL IRREGULARITY AND FACIAL PLETHORA 7

SUMMARY OF URINE STEROID STUDIES

DAY	17-OHCS	Free Cortisol
Baseline	11 mg/gm Cr	89 µg/gm Cr
Dexamethasone 2 mg (2nd day)	9 mg/gm Cr	89 µg/gm Cr
Dexamethasone 8 mg (2nd day)	2.1 mg/gm Cr	24 µg/gm Cr

Since you now know the most likely source of hyper-cortisolism in this patient is the pituitary, you <u>order an enhanced computerized tomography (CT) scan of the pituitary</u>. *[The CT scan was normal.]* At some centers bilateral simultaneous venous catheterization of inferior petrosal veins measuring ACTH gradients helps to localize the tumor. *[It was not performed in this patient.]* Also, one always has to worry about the rare ectopic and usually indolent tumor (e.g., bronchial carcinoid) that mimics pituitary adenoma. A <u>chest X-ray</u> and often a <u>chest CT</u> are indicated.

What about a CT scan of the adrenals? Although one could argue fiscally that this is not necessary in this patient, a CT scan was obtained and demonstrated equal size adrenals which were questionably enlarged. <u>The clinical diagnosis is Cushing's disease</u>.

4. <u>Transsphenoidal pituitary microsurgery (TPS)</u>, which can cure 85-95% of patients while preserving pituitary function, is the therapy of choice for Cushing's disease. However, these impressive results are not obtained in all centers, and therefore, the choice of treatment between TPS and bilateral adrenalectomy will vary. Cyproheptadine, metyrapone, or ketoconazole has occasionally produced amelioration of symptoms, but the results are generally poor.

5. TPS often cures the hypercortisolism and restores pituitary function. <u>You need the results of TPS at your institution</u> That depends on the skill of the neurosurgeon, the size of the adenoma (whether it can be found), and whether total or subtotal hypophysectomy is performed if the adenoma is not

8   CASE STUDIES IN ENDOCRINOLOGY

identified. The cure rate ranges from 10-95%. If bilateral adrenalectomy is advised, then the patient will be permanently dependent on replacement glucocorticoid and mineralocorticoid. Significant hyperpigmentation and sella enlargement due to a large ACTH-producing tumor (Nelson's syndrome) follow adrenalectomy in about 8% (range, 5-35%) of cases.

PEARLS:

1. The most common cause of Cushing's syndrome remains iatrogenic—taking glucocorticoids in pharmacologic doses for nonendocrine disease (includes absorption of topical steroids). Surreptitious abuse of steroids should also be considered.

2. One of the best ways to make the diagnosis of Cushing's syndrome is by comparing photographs of the patient taken over the previous years. Arranging these snapshots (driver's license, class photographs, etc.) chronologically aids in making the diagnosis.

3. Although the diurnal pattern of plasma cortisol is often lost in Cushing's disease, the comparison of 7-8 AM to 4-6 PM plasma cortisol levels is not helpful diagnostically. There is too much variation within the normal ranges at these times. A more specific study would be to obtain blood late at night between 11 PM and 1 AM. The plasma cortisol should be < 5 µg/dl in normal non-stressed individuals. In 95% of patients with endogenous hypercortisolism, the late night cortisol will be > 5 µg/dl.

MENSTRUAL IRREGULARITY AND FACIAL PLETHORA 9

4. Children and young adults often do not have hypertension with Cushing's syndrome. However, <u>hypertension nearly always accompanies hypercortisolism after the age of 40.</u>

5. <u>The CT scan of the pituitary rarely shows any abnormality in Cushing's disease.</u> The adenoma is small, typically < 5 mm.

6. <u>Immediate hypoadrenalism following TPS in Cushing's disease is the best prognostic sign for cure.</u> The patient may remain hypoadrenal for months before the normal pituitary-adrenal axis recovers from chronic glucocorticoid suppression.

7. ACTH levels fall within the normal range (20-80 pg/ml) in at least half of the patients with Cushing's disease. Nonmeasurable ACTH levels in patients with Cushing's syndrome suggest adrenal adenoma/carcinoma (one must consider exogenous intake of glucocorticoids as well). ACTH levels > 200 pg/ml usually mean ectopic ACTH syndrome.

8. Ectopic ACTH syndrome presents with a different picture than classical Cushing's syndrome. The patients are often older men (age, 50-70 years) who present with severe weakness, weight loss, and metabolic hypokalemic alkalosis without the physical stigmata of chronic hypercortisolism seen the young women (20-40 years) with Cushing's disease. <u>Oat cell carcinoma of the lung is the most frequent cause of ectopic ACTH syndrome.</u>

PITFALLS:

1. Often we present and describe the patient at the bedside. Be sensitive and avoid using terms such as "moon facies," "buffalo hump," "dewlap," etc.

10   CASE STUDIES IN ENDOCRINOLOGY

2. Failure of the AM plasma cortisol to suppress after giving dexamethasone 1 mg at bedtime does not mean that the patient has hypercortisolism. Any form of stress (e.g., failure to get a good night's sleep, severe illness, surgery, trauma, fever, infection, dehydration, alcoholism, depression) may prevent pituitary-adrenal suppression to this dose of dexamethasone. Taking phenytoin or phenobarbital increases dexamethasone degradation so sufficient serum dexamethasone levels may not develop, leading to nonsuppressed cortisol levels. Furthermore, women taking oral contraceptives may not suppress their AM cortisol since estrogens stimulate synthesis of cortisol binding globulin, the major plasma protein on which cortisol circulates.

3. ACTH levels may help in diagnosing the etiology of the hypercortisolism, but proper handling of the specimen is critical. ACTH adheres to glass avidly. Blood must be collected in heparin or EDTA tubes, and plasma must be separated immediately at 4°C and then stored frozen in plastic tubes. If handling is careless, any interpretation of ACTH values is meaningless. In addition, ACTH should be measured by a laboratory that has much experience with ACTH determinations.

4. Always interpret urine 17-OHCS collections using urine creatinine as the measure of adequacy of collection. Expressing the data in milligrams of 17-OHCS/grams of creatinine gives fewer false positive results than expressing data in milligrams of 17-OHCS/24 hours.

5. Care should be taken to make sure the patient is not taking any medication during the 24-hour urine collection for 17-OHCS. At least 30 commonly prescribed drugs may interfere with the 17-OHCS determination (a colorimetric assay).

MENSTRUAL IRREGULARITY AND FACIAL PLETHORA 11

6. Although administrating corticotropin releasing factor (CRF) to stimulate ACTH may serve to differentiate between the types of Cushing's syndrome, its usefulness is limited by the availability of CRF and the problems that come with measurement of ACTH.

REFERENCES

Aron DC, Findling JW, Fitzgerald PA, et al: Cushing's syndrome: problems in management. Endocr Rev 3: 229, 1982.

Aron DC, Tyrrell JB, Fitzgerald PA, et al: Cushing's syndrome: problems in diagnosis. Medicine 60: 25, 1981.

Burch W: A survey of results with transsphenoidal surgery in Cushing's disease. N Engl J Med 308:103, 1983.

Burch WM: Cushing's disease: a review. Arch Intern Med 145:1106, 1985.

Carpenter PC: Cushing's syndrome: update of diagnosis and management. Mayo Clin Proc 61:49, 1986.

Kreiger DT. Physiopathology of Cushing's disease. Endocr Rev 4:22, 1983.

Liddle GW: Tests of pituitary adrenal suppressibility in the diagnosis of Cushing's syndrome. J Clin Endocrinol Metab 20:1539, 1960.

Sindler BH, Griffing GT, Melby JC: The superiority of the metyrapone test versus the high-dose dexamethasone test in the differential diagnosis of Cushing's syndrome. Am J Med 74:657, 1983.

Tyrrell JB, Findling JW, Aron DC, et al: An overnight high-dose dexamethasone suppression test for rapid differential diagnosis of Cushing's syndrome. Ann Intern Med 104:180, 1986.

PERSISTENT HYPOKALEMIA

CASE 2: J.W., a 45-year-old farmer, presented with a 2-week history of proximal muscle weakness. He described this weakness as not being able to raise his arms to comb his hair and an inability to stoop. His review of systems was negative for alcohol use, nocturia, polyuria, recent weight change, headache, chest pain, or diarrhea. Past medical history was significant for hypertension of 5 years' duration treated with hydrochlorothiazide, KCl, prazosin, and propranolol. He had been told that he had "a low blood chemical due to his medications" for which KCl had been prescribed. There was no family history of weakness, but both of his parents took antihypertensive medication.

On examination, he was a plethoric, obese, white male weighing 200 lb (height, 68 inches; pulse, 68 and regular; afebrile). His BP was 180/120 sitting and standing. Eye exam revealed normal optic disks, mild arteriolar-venous nicking, and no retinal hemorrhages or exudates. Thyroid was not palpable. An S4 was present on cardiac exam. He had a protuberant abdomen without hepatosplenomegaly and normal genitalia. There was no centripetal obesity. The skin showed no striae. Neurological exam revealed decreased girdle strength 4/5. Mental status, sensory, deep tendon reflexes, and cerebellar exams were normal.

ENDOCRINE CLUE: An ECG was obtained.

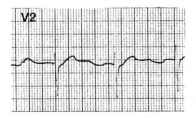 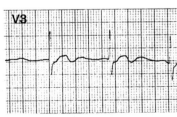

PERSISTENT HYPOKALEMIA 13

Note the prominent U waves, suggesting hypokalemia or hypocalcemia. Since the Q-T interval was not prolonged, you make a tentative diagnosis of hypokalemia and order the following studies.

Serum electrolytes: Na, 143 mEq/l; K, 2.0 mEq/l; HCO_3, 34 mEq/l; Cl, 106 mEq/l; BUN, 14 mg/dl; Cr, 1.1 mg/dl. Serum Ca was 8.9 mg/dl; P, 3.6 mg/dl; albumin, 4.0 mg/dl. Serum creatine phosphokinase (CPK): 5700 U/l (normal, < 120).

QUESTIONS:

1. What problems might cause the elevated serum CPK in this patient? Which is most likely?

2. What further studies would you recommend to evaluate the serum potassium and CPK?

3. He was treated with prazosin and KCl for 4 weeks (previous meds were discontinued). He returned and his BP was 170/105, serum K was 2.6 mEq/l, and the serum CPK was 105 U/l. What would you do now?

4. After a review of the studies performed in Question #3, what is this patient's diagnosis?

5. How would you manage this problem?

14   CASE STUDIES IN ENDOCRINOLOGY

ANSWERS:

1. The most likely source of CPK in this patient with weakness is muscle. Any process which causes increased CPK release (e.g., muscle destruction) or decreased clearance of CPK (e.g., hypothyroidism) might raise serum CPK levels. Hypokalemia and muscle weakness suggest <u>periodic paralysis</u>, but the magnitude of the CPK elevation points to a muscle destruction that might be seen with <u>polymyositis or rhabdomyolysis</u>. Since hypokalemia may cause rhabdomyolysis, the most likely cause of weakness is <u>hypokalemic-induced rhabdomyolysis</u>.

2. To confirm the rhabdomyolysis, <u>check the urine for myoglobin</u>. *[The urine had a pink color; the lab confirmed myoglobinuria.]* The hypokalemia needs evaluation. Most likely, the hypokalemia reflects loss of potassium via the urine or GI tract. Taking diuretics for hypertension causes most hypokalemia and should be considered first in this patient. <u>Stopping the diuretic is obvious</u>. An ECG is necessary to monitor rhythm and check for myocardial injury. Prominent U waves should decrease as the serum K rises. You should <u>collect a 24-hour urine and measure the urine potassium</u>. If the urine contains < 30 mEq K/day, then the hypokalemia reflects loss of prior diuretic therapy or GI loss. If the urine contains > 40 mEq/day, then renal wasting of K is confirmed. Because of the possibility that hypokalemia caused his weakness, this patient was treated with KCl initially, so a 24-hour urine for K was not collected. However, the possibility of Cushing's syndrome (hypertension, obesity, and facial plethora) warrants a <u>24-hour collection for 17-OHCS and/or free cortisol</u>. *[His urine 17-OHCS level was 3.0 mg/gm creatinine (normal).]* Within 3 days, his CPK was normal and the serum potassium rose to 3.2 mEq/l on a sodium restricted diet.

PERSISTENT HYPOKALEMIA   15

3. <u>Spontaneous hypokalemia in a hypertensive patient means mineralocorticoid excess until proved otherwise.</u> Obtaining a <u>plasma renin</u> helps define whether the mineralocorticoid excess is secondary (activated renin-angiotensin system as in volume contraction, renovascular hypertension, estrogen-induced hypertension from increased renin substrate, or malignant hypertension) or is primary (primary aldosteronism or pseudoaldosteronism as in licorice ingestion or excess of other mineralocorticoids). *[Plasma renin activity (PRA) was low, suggesting mineralocorticoid excess.]* Any hyperkalemic, hypertensive patient needs to be asked about licorice ingestion. *[He denied taking licorice containing candies, drinks, or tobacco products; PRA is low in licorice abuse as well.]* <u>Measuring a 24-hour urine for aldosterone and potassium</u> is the next step in a patient who has low renin hypertension and spontaneous hypokalemia. *[Urine K was 85 mEq/day and urine aldosterone levels were elevated.]*

4. <u>Primary hyperaldosteronism.</u> Most patients (65-85%) have an <u>aldosterone-producing adrenal adenoma (APA)</u> as the source of the hyperaldosteronism; the remainder have idiopathic hyperaldosteronism as bilateral adrenal hyperplasia (15-35%). Very rarely adrenal carcinoma presents with hypokalemia (17-ketosteroids are high and an abdominal mass usually evident).

5. Successful management depends on resolving whether the hyperaldosteronism results from an aldosteronoma (APA) or bilateral adrenal hyperplasia. Removing the aldosteronoma cures the hypokalemia and in least 85% of patients abolishes the hypertension. <u>Surgical extirpation for bilateral adrenal hyperplasia rarely cures the hypertension and leaves the patients dependent on steroid replacement for the remainder of their life.</u>

Several methods have been proposed to differentiate between APA and bilateral adrenal hyperplasia. <u>Order CT scan of the adrenals</u>. CT scanning of the adrenals is helpful when both adrenals are visualized and there is clearly a mass in one adrenal. Unfortunately, that circumstance is not common because most aldosteronomas are < 2 cm in size, and thus are below the resolution of many scanners. *[Adrenal CT showed no abnormality in this patient.]* Provocative studies such as aldosterone response to upright posture, furosemide, or captopril have been used to aid localization. <u>The most accurate study in the differential diagnosis of primary aldosteronism is bilateral adrenal vein sampling for measurement of aldosterone/cortisol ratios performed by an experienced angiographer.</u> Aldosterone levels from an aldosteronoma are least 10 times higher than those from the contralateral adrenal. *[Adrenal vein catheterization was performed and an aldosterone of gradient of 20:1 (right versus left adrenal vein) was found.]* Surgery via a posterior incision on the right flank through the bed of the 12th rib was performed. The photograph shows the tumor within the adrenal. Note a small round lesion (*arrow*) that was characteristically yellow on sectioning. Again, CT scanning did not help in this patient.

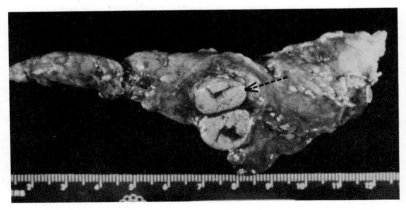

PERSISTENT HYPOKALEMIA 17

PEARLS:

1. Unmeasurable plasma renin activity in a patient receiving diuretics is strong evidence for primary aldosteronism.

2. Most hypertensive patients with spontaneous hypokalemia have primary hyperaldosteronism.

3. The degree of hypokalemia in primary aldosteronism depends on sodium intake. Salt restriction leads to potassium retention and ameliorates the hypokalemia. Likewise, sodium loading may exacerbate the hypokalemia and accentuate the hypokalemic manifestations, causing more weakness and possibly perilous cardiac problems.

4. If the serum potassium remains normal in a patient who has normal renal function and who ingests generous quantities of sodium (> 100 mEq/day) while not taking potassium-sparing diuretics, primary aldosteronism is effectively excluded.

5. If the CT shows an adrenal mass in a patient who has been diagnosed as having primary aldosteronism, then further workup may be avoided, and the patient may be assumed to have an aldosterone-producing adenoma.

6. Spironolactone (up to 200 mg twice a day) or amiloride (10-40 mg each day) is used to treat patients with idiopathic hyperaldosteronism or in those patients with APA who refuse surgery. Gynecomastia and impotence are the major side effects of spironolactone treatment.

7. Licorice ingestion may mimic hyperaldosteronism. However, plasma and urine aldosterone levels are low. Patient who chew tobacco heavily flavored with licorice and who swallow the saliva are at risk for pseudoaldosteronism. Most licorice

flavoring is artificial and does not contain the active component, glycyrrhizinic acid, which causes hypertension.

8. The following algorithm helps evaluate the hypertensive patient with hypokalemia.

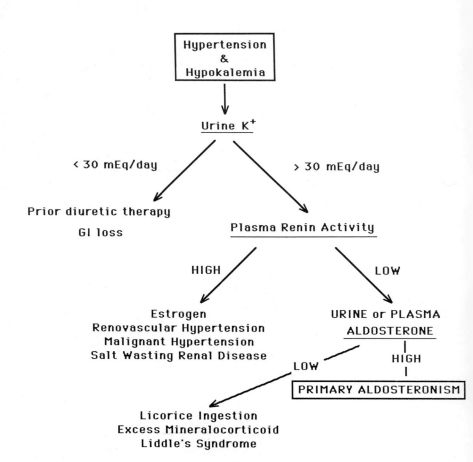

PITFALLS:

1. Decreased plasma renin activity is found in 20% of the hypertensive population. Thus, a low renin value alone is not of much help.

2. Although plasma aldosterone levels are high and plasma renin activity low in primary aldosteronism, plasma aldosterone levels may be normal, particularly after noon in patients with primary aldosteronism. That is why studies taken in the morning and then several hours later must be interpreted with care (circadian variation in plasma aldosterone occurs in APA).

3. Avoid giving sodium to a hypokalemic patient who you suspect might have primary aldosteronism. You might precipitate hypokalemic crisis.

4. Often the right adrenal vein is difficult to catheterize, and thus adrenal venous sampling to differentiate APA from idiopathic hyperaldosteronism may not be as helpful as one might like. If, however, the right adrenal vein is entered, the accuracy of comparative adrenal aldosterone level in diagnosing APA or bilateral adrenal hyperplasia exceeds 95%.

5. Saline infusion (2 liters over 4 hours) provides a rapid outpatient method to test for primary aldosteronism. The diagnosis is confirmed if plasma aldosterone levels fail to fall below 10 ng/dl. The test relies on single plasma aldosterone level (a potential problem) and should not be done in patients with severe hypertension and compensated congestive heart failure.

6. Do not forget to ask about nasal sprays and topical creams in patients who may have chronic rhinitis or sinusitis. Habitual

20 CASE STUDIES IN ENDOCRINOLOGY

use of 9-alpha-fluoroprednisolone and other vasoconstrictor agents may mimic hyperaldosteronism.

REFERENCES

Alder GK, Williams GH: Primary aldosteronism. In Krieger DT, Bardin CW (eds): Current Therapy in Endocrinology and Metabolism 1985-1986.Toronto, B.C. Decker, 1985, pp 116-121.

Arteaga E, Klein R, Biglieri EG: Use of the saline infusion test to diagnose the cause of primary aldosteronism. Am J Med 79:722, 1985.

Battle DC, Kurtzman NA: Clinical disorders of aldosterone metabolism. DM 30:1-55, 1984.

Blachley JD, Knochel JP: Tobacco chewer's hypokalemia: licorice revisited. N Engl J Med 302:784, 1980.

Conn JW, Cohen EL, Rovner DR: Landmark article: suppression of plasma renin activity in primary aldosteronism. JAMA 253:558, 1985.

Conn JW, Rovner DR, Cohen EL: Licorice-induced pseudoaldosteronism. JAMA 205:80, 1968.

Grant CS, Carpenter PC, van Heerden JA, et al: Primary aldosteronism. Arch Surg 119:585, 1984.

Kaplan NM: Endocrine hypertension. In Wilson JD, Foster DW (eds): Textbook of Endocrinology, ed. 7. Philadelphia, W.B. Saunders, 1985, pp 966-988.

Melby JC: Primary aldosteronism. Kidney Int 26:769, 1984.

Weinberger MH: Primary aldosteronism: diagnosis and differentiation of types. Ann Intern Med 100:300, 1984.

INCIDENTAL ADRENAL MASS

CASE 3: L.K., a 30-year-old grocery clerk, presented for evaluation of hematuria. He had been in excellent health until he awoke with severe right flank pain associated with red colored urine. The pain radiated to his right groin. He had no previous history of kidney stones or genitourinary infection. His father and paternal uncle had passed stones in their urine. There was no family history of gout.

Physical exam revealed a healthy appearing white male in moderate distress. Vital signs: BP, 130/80 mm Hg; pulse, 95/min; temperature, 37°C; weight, 165 lb; height, 70 inches. The only remarkable finding was right flank tenderness.

ENDOCRINE CLUE: Urine analysis: red tinged; many erythrocytes (too numerous to count); trace protein; negative glucose; urine culture, pending. An intravenous pyelogram was ordered. The right ureter had a small filling defect which did not totally obstruct the flow of contrast media. Because a questionable left suprarenal mass, CT of the abdomen was ordered.

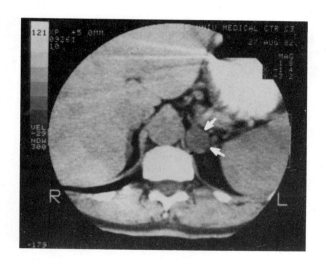

QUESTIONS:

1. What does the CT scan show?

2. What is the differential diagnosis for such a finding?

3. What further studies are indicated for this patient?

4. What are useful CT criteria in evaluating patients with this problem?

5. After gathering the data ordered, what would you recommend to this patient?

24   CASE STUDIES IN ENDOCRINOLOGY

ANSWERS:

1. The CT scan shows a 3-cm mass in the left adrenal gland. The mass does not enhance with contrast medium and appears homogeneous with well-defined margins. Thus, an adrenal mass is found incidentally on CT scan.

2. Although it is unlikely that the adrenal mass pertains to the patient's current problem, several possibilities need to be excluded. Unilateral masses within the adrenal include functioning or nonfunctioning tumors that may be benign or malignant. Nonfunctioning adrenal tumors are common. Clinically silent tumors occur in 1.4 to 8.7% of autopsied patients. Such tumors include benign cortical adenomas, cysts, myelolipomas, ganglioneuromas, hemorrhages, and granulomas. Malignant nonfunctioning masses include metastatic tumors and adrenal adenocarcinomas which are often bulky tumors (> 6 cm). Functioning tumors include cortical adenomas that secrete cortisol (Cushing's syndrome), androgens (virilizing syndromes), aldosterone (Conn's syndrome), and medullary adenomas that secrete catecholamines (pheochromocytoma). Histologically, these tumors are generally benign.

3. The working diagnosis is nephrolithiasis and an incidental adrenal mass. Order a serum calcium and phosphorus to check for hyperparathyroidism. *[Ca, 9.4 mg/dl; P, 3.7 mg/dl; the serum uric acid was 4.0 mg/dl.]* Order serum electrolytes, BUN, and creatinine to assess renal function. *[All were normal; specifically K, 4.0 mEq/l]*. Urine studies that may prove helpful include 24-hour collections for calcium, oxalate, and uric acid.

   You must ask yourself whether the adrenal mass is a functioning or a nonfunctioning tumor. If it is a functioning

INCIDENTAL ADRENAL MASS   25

endocrine tumor, surgical removal is necessary. Use the following table to help you rule out a functioning tumor.

Possibility	Order
Cushing's syndrome	24-hour urine for 17-OHCS/UC; (dexamethasone study if urine abnormal or if you suspect Cushing's syndrome clinically)
Virilizing syndrome	24-hour urine for 17-KS, 17-OHCS; (serum testosterone, serum 17-OHCS if hirsute female; serum estrogen for feminized male or child)
Aldosteronoma	Serum potassium on high sodium diet (200 mEq or more); if low (< 3.5) or patient hypertensive, measure 24-hour urine aldosterone
Pheochromocytoma	24-hour urine for vanillylmandelic acid or metanephrine or catecholamines (get two different studies if patient hypertensive)

If the tumor is nonfunctioning, use the CT criteria given below to help you decide what to do.

4. The CT scan gives you hints as to whether the mass is benign or malignant. Three criteria are important: size, contrast enhancement, and consistency. Malignant adenocarcinomas are large (in six series, 105 out of 114 adenocarcinomas were 6 cm or greater). Benign adenomas rarely get this size (3 out 12,000 autopsies). So any mass > 6 cm ought to be removed. For the majority of adrenal masses (i.e., nonfunctioning masses < 6 cm in size), contrast enhancement and consistency help with the probability of malignancy. Contrast

26 CASE STUDIES IN ENDOCRINOLOGY

enhancement is more often seen in malignant lesions. Benign adrenal lesions generally have a regular consistency (homogeneous appearance on CT), whereas malignant lesions show irregular consistency (hypodense and soft tissue mixed haphazardly).

It is possible to estimate the probability of malignancy using these criteria (data of Hussain et al.) Note: This data was drawn from functioning and nonfunctioning tumors.

	PROBABILTY of MALIGNANCY	
SIZE (cm)	No Enhancement	Enhancement
2.0	0.14	0.43
3.0	0.18	0.52
4.0	0.24	0.60
5.0	0.31	0.68
6.0	0.39	0.75
7.0	0.47	0.81
8.0	0.56	0.86

5. For the nephrolithiasis, he spontaneously passed a stone (analyzed to be calcium oxalate). This type of stone and family history suggest absorptive hypercalciuria. Good hydration, particularly at bedtime (drinking 8 ounces or more of water), might help prevent recurrence. If stones do recur, hypercalciuria should be documented and treated with thiazide diuretics.

For the patient's incidental adrenal mass, the endocrine studies found nothing to suggest that this was a functioning adenoma (requiring surgery). The CT parameters suggested that this was a benign lesion. In the event that this might be a small nonfunctioning adenocarcinoma, CT in 6 months and at 12 months should be performed. If the left adrenal enlarges, then adrenalectomy is in order. If unchanged in size, it is

INCIDENTAL ADRENAL MASS 27

unlikely to be malignant. Follow-up CT scanning seems nonproductive in the latter instance.

PEARLS:

1. The CT has made incidentally discovered adrenal mass (adrenal "incidentaloma") a real clinical problem. In approaching this problem, first determine whether the mass is hormonally active (see Answer #3). If so, then surgical extirpation is necessary. For nonfunctioning complex masses > 6 cm, surgery is again indicated. For nonfunctioning masses larger than > 6 cm that appear totally cystic, then fine needle aspiration might be attempted.

2. For small adrenal "incidentalomas" (nonfunctioning and < 6 cm which appear homogeneous on CT scan), follow-up CT scans in 6 and 12 months seem reasonable.

3. Adrenal adenocarcinomas are generally large, palpable tumors that do not secrete much cortisol. Thus, these patients may not appear Cushingoid. However, secretion of precursors of cortisol is often high, leading to hirsutism and/or virilization. Urine 17-ketosteroids (17-KS) levels may be astronomical. When the 17-KS values are higher than the 17-OHCS values, think adrenal carcinoma.

4. The cortisol-secreting adenoma is the most common functioning adrenal tumor. However, these patients are not truly asymptomatic (i.e., do not qualify as an "incidentaloma").

5. Among 51 reported adrenal "incidentalomas" found by CT, 3 had unsuspected pheochromocytomas while the rest were causes where surgical intervention would not be necessary.

28   CASE STUDIES IN ENDOCRINOLOGY

PITFALLS:

1. Calcifications within an adrenal mass do not point to a benign or malignant process.

2. Angiography is not sufficiently specific to diagnose the cause of an adrenal mass.

3. Fine needle aspiration of adrenal lesions has limited usefulness. The cytopathology will not distinguish between benign and malignant tumors. Large cysts can, however, be drained. Clear fluid is uniformly associated with benign processes whereas bloody fluid may be associated with benign or malignant processes.

REFERENCES

Case records of the Massachusetts General Hospital. Weekly clinicopathological exercises. Case 38-1984: hypertension and an adrenal mass after a vehicular accident. N Engl J Med 311:783, 1984.

Copeland PM: The incidentally discovered adrenal mass. Ann Intern Med 98:940, 1983.

Guerrero LA: Diagnostic and therapeutic approach to incidental adrenal mass. Urology 26:435, 1985.

Hussain S, Belldegrun A, Seltzer SE, et al: Differentiation of malignant from benign adrenal masses: Predictive indices on computed tomography. AJR 144:61, 1985.

Moore MA, Biggs PJ: Unilateral adrenal hemorrhage: an unusual presentation. South Med J 78:989, 1985.

SPELLS

CASE 4: R.D., a 36-year-old unemployed man, presents for the evaluation of "spells." For the last 3 years, he has experienced episodes that occur during jogging. After running 1 mile, he feels dizzy and lightheaded and has a headache that lasts for 5-10 minutes. These episodes occurred infrequently until about a year ago, and now occur several times a week and not only during jogging. A typical episode begins with dizziness, followed by tremulous hands and a sensation that his face is pale. He feels his heart pounding but has not noticed an increase in heart rate. When the episodes are more severe, the above symptoms are followed by perspiration and headache over the nuchal area. These spells last from 5-30 minutes, leaving him weak and tired. His general health has been excellent. He has seen several physicians (including a psychiatrist) for these spells. Many studies, including an oral glucose tolerance test (looking for reactive hypoglycemia) and an exercise treadmill ECG (looking for arrhythmias), failed to identify a specific cause. His social history reveals that he had been a marketing manager (moved to a new area but the job did not work out) and now is in his second marriage. His wife is employed, and he has been sitting around the house writing resumes for other jobs. He denies impotence or weight loss. No family history of diabetes mellitus or other endocrine disease is elicited; his father died of lymphosarcoma.

The physical exam is entirely normal (BP, 124/82; pulse, 78/min; weight, 181 lb; height, 71 inches). He is a pleasant white male who is not particularly anxious. His affect and mental status exam seem normal. The skin reveals no areas of hyperpigmentation. No masses are palpable in the neck.

30   CASE STUDIES IN ENDOCRINOLOGY

ENDOCRINE CLUE: Since the spells were often related to exercise, you ask him to do 50 jumping jacks. Immediately after he finishes, his pulse is regular at 125/min and BP 180/100. No typical spell is induced. His BP 10 minutes later is 145/90.

SPELLS   31

QUESTIONS:

1. What are the possible diagnoses?

2. What studies would you order?

3. Some of the studies you requested were abnormal (Question #2). What would you do to follow up this result?

4. What is the diagnosis?

5. How would you manage this patient?

32   CASE STUDIES IN ENDOCRINOLOGY

ANSWERS:

1. The nonspecificity of his complaints opens a Pandora's box of possible diagnoses. His symptoms are that of increased adrenergic discharge. Given his social history, the most likely cause is chronic anxiety/stress syndrome. Other diagnoses include "reactive" hypoglycemia (akin to anxiety), hyperthyroidism (accentuates sympathetic tone), and catecholamine-secreting tumors. His story is compatible with a pheochromocytoma. The persistent elevation of his blood pressure after exercise should make you suspicious.

2. Hyperthyroidism (though unlikely) could be ruled out by ordering a serum T4 and T3U. *[T4, 8.9 µg/dl; T3U, 40% (normal, 35-45%.]* A 24-hour urine for vanillylmandelic acid (VMA), metanephrines, or catecholamines should be collected to check the possibility of a pheochromocytoma. Each of these measurements is equally useful. Plasma catecholamine levels are helpful under research conditions, but urine determinations are superior and more specific in making the diagnosis of pheochromocytoma. In patients who have a strong clinical suspicion of a catecholamine-producing tumor, the author prefers to get two different determinations on the same collection. *[VMA, 13.8 mg/gm creatinine (normal, < 7 mg/gm).]* You are surprised and order catecholamines on the same urine. *[Epinephrine, 450 µg/24 hours; norepinephrine, 220 µg/24 hours (normal, < 100 µg/24 hours each).]*

3. The diagnosis of pheochromocytoma is likely. To localize the tumor, you go back and carefully palpate the neck and order a chest X-ray. Ninety-eight percent of pheochromocytomas are within the abdomen; the others are found in the posterior mediastinum or are readily palpable as a carotid body tumor. Abdominal CT facilitates the localization of the tumor. *[On CT scan, this patient's left adrenal contained a 4-cm mass.]*

SPELLS 33

4. The preoperative diagnosis was <u>pheochromocytoma</u>. You order blood for <u>serum calcium and calcitonin determinations</u> to rule out the remote possibility of multiple endocrine neoplasia (MEN).

5. <u>The treatment is surgical removal of the left adrenal gland.</u> Preoperative management includes alpha-adrenergic blockade using phenoxybenzamine in an initial dose of 10 mg three times a day. The dose may need to be increased over several days (up to 40 mg three times a day) until the blood pressure stabilizes in hypertensive patients, symptoms abate, and hypovolemia remits. This patient did not need propranolol. Intraoperative management requires expert anesthesia care. Intravenous phentolamine or nitroprusside is used to treat acute hypertensive episodes. Propranolol or lidocaine may be used to manage cardiac arrhythmias. The entire abdomen needs to be explored to search for multiple tumors along the aortic chain.

PEARLS:

1. The diagnosis of pheochromocytoma cannot be made on clinical grounds alone. <u>The suspicion of a catecholamine-producing tumor is raised in a hypertensive patient who has spells with sweating, headache, and palpitations</u>. The diagnosis requires biochemical evidence of increased catecholamine secretion.

2. Sustained hypertension is the rule in most patients with pheochromocytoma; hypertension that is episodic and severe is less common. However, even in the patient with sustained hypertension, wide fluctuations and paroxysmal increases in blood pressure might alert you to the possibility of pheochromocytoma.

34   CASE STUDIES IN ENDOCRINOLOGY

3. The clinical features in patients with pheochromocytoma depend upon the predominant catecholamine secreted. Norepinephrine-producing tumors (the most common type) have hypertension as the primary manifestation. If these tumors secrete significant amounts of epinephrine, then sweating, nervousness, and palpitations are present. A pure epinephrine-secreting tumor is rare (marked by tachycardia, hypertension, and postural hypotension and found exclusively in the adrenals).

4. A family history of pheochromocytoma should be sought. About 10% of cases of pheochromocytoma occur as simple familial pheochromocytoma or as part of the multiple endocrine neoplasia syndrome (MEN type IIa or IIb).

5. Metaiodobenzylguanidine (MIBG) is trapped by neural crest tissue. Scintiscan using radiolabeled I-131-MIBG helps localize disease in patients who have multiple pheochromocytomas or who have recurrent disease following surgery. Large doses of I-131-MIBG can be used to treat metastatic pheochromocytoma.

6. Patients with familial pheochromocytoma are younger than the sporadic cases and often have bilateral adrenal and extra-adrenal sites of disease. <u>Neurofibromatosis and cafe-au-lait spots should be sought</u>.

PITFALLS:

1. Provocative testing with agents such as tyramine, histamine, or glucagon is not advised. <u>The results are unreliable and the hazards related to the testing are substantial</u>.

SPELLS 35

2. Most patients with pheochromocytoma have no clinical evidence for hyperparathyroidism or medullary thyroid carcinoma. However, since the patient with pheochromocytoma might have an unrecognized MEN (type II) syndrome, <u>serum calcium and calcitonin measurements should be determined</u>.

3. If beta-blocking drugs such as propranolol are used prior to surgery for pheochromocytoma, alpha-adrenergic blockade should be started <u>first</u>, then the beta-blocker. Beta-blockade alone may worsen the hypertension and aggravate the tachycardia.

REFERENCES

Cryer PE: Diseases of the adrenal medullae and sympathetic nervous system. In Felig P, Baxter JD, Broadus AE, Frohman LA (eds): <u>Endocrinology and Metabolism</u>. New York, McGraw-Hill, 1981, pp 511-550.

Gilford RW Jr, Bravo EL, Manger WM: Diagnosis and management of pheochromocytoma. <u>Cardiology</u> 72:Suppl 1, 126, 1985.

Gough IR, Thompson NW, Shapiro B, Sisson JC: Limitations of 131I-MIBG scintigraphy in locating pheochromocytomas. <u>Surgery</u> 98:115, 1985.

Levine SN, McDonald JC: The evaluation and management of pheochromocytomas. <u>Adv Surg</u> 17:281, 1984.

Shapiro B, Sisson JC, Eyre P, et al: 131I-MIBG: a new agent in the diagnosis and treatment of pheochromocytoma. <u>Cardiology</u> 72:Suppl 1, 137, 1985.

Sjoerdsma A, Engelman K, Waldman TA, et al: Pheochromocytoma: current concepts of diagnosis and treatment. <u>Ann Intern Med</u> 65:1302, 1966.

SEVERE WEAKNESS AND RECTAL BLEEDING

CASE 5: G.R., a 50-year-old homemaker, was admitted to the hospital because of rectal bleeding. For last 3 months she had experienced a 8-lb weight loss and progressive weakness so that she could walk no more than 100 feet without having to sit down. When she saw her physician, she denied any dyspnea, cough, polyuria, or use of any medications. Her physical exam was reported as normal. Laboratory studies are given in the CLUE. One week later she returned, stating that she had two bowel movements that morning which were grossly bloody, and she was admitted to the hospital. There was no history of abdominal pain, diarrhea, constipation, hemorrhoids, diabetes, or hypertension. She did not smoke tobacco or abuse alcohol.

On examination, the BP was 150/95 mm Hg lying, 140/85 standing; pulse, 90/min; weight, 120 lb; height, 65 inches. She was an alert white female who appeared in no acute distress. Mental status exam was normal. She had a ruddy complexion, several ecchymoses (2 x 2 cm) over the lower extremities, and normal skin texture without hirsutism. HEENT, thyroid, chest, and heart exams were normal. The liver span was 12 cm and the margin of the liver was palpable 3 cm below right midcostal margin. No hepatic nodules were identified. The reminder of the abdominal exam and pelvic exam were normal. No masses were found on rectal exam. The stool was trace positive for occult blood. Neurologic exam showed promixal muscular weakness (she could not stand up from a squatting position). Deep tendon reflexes were normal.

ENDOCRINE CLUE: Hemoglobin, 13.5 gm/dl; hemocrit, 38%. Serum electrolytes: Na, 138 mEq/l, K, 2.9 mEq/l, HCO_3 30 mEq/l; Cl, 100 mEq/l; plasma glucose, 200 mg/dl; BUN, 10 mg/dl; Ca, 9.5 mg/dl; and T4(RIA), 7.0 µg/dl.

QUESTIONS:

1. What is the differential diagnosis?

2. What further studies are indicated?

3. Given the results in Question #2, what is the most likely diagnosis?

4. What would you recommend next?

5. What is the treatment for this condition?

38 CASE STUDIES IN ENDOCRINOLOGY

ANSWERS:

1. The causes of weight loss are numerous. Diagnoses to be considered in this patient include diabetes mellitus (elevated plasma glucose), malabsorption (enteritis with hemorrhage), hyperadrenalism (raised BP, ecchymosis, elevated plasma glucose, hypokalemia), or cancer (hepatomegaly, bowel lesion with hemorrhage, ectopic ACTH secretion, and the remote effects of carcinoma). Hyperthyroidism seems unlikely with a normal serum T4 and pulse rate and the absence of thyromegaly.

2. The combination of weight loss, weakness, hypokalemia, and alkalosis suggests ectopic ACTH syndrome. To address the hypercortisolism, you ask for a 24-hour urine for 17-OHCS and/or free cortisol and a plasma ACTH level. Knowing that the most common source of ectopic ACTH syndrome is small cell carcinoma of the lung, you order a chest X-ray. *[Chest X-ray, normal.]* To address the hematochezia, sigmoidoscopic exam was performed. *[No lesions identified; stool now negative.]* Because of the hepatomegaly, you order SGOT, SGPT, bilirubin, alkaline phosphatase, and liver radionuclide scan. *[The biochemical studies were normal; liver scan showed three focal areas of decreased uptake.]* Five days later, the 17-OHCS returned at 25 mg/gm creatinine (normal, < 6.5) and ACTH at 1200 pg/ml (normal, 20-80).

3. High plasma ACTH level, increased urine 17-OHCS, and hypodense liver densities point to ectopic ACTH syndrome. The autonomy of cortisol secretion was confirmed with dexamethasone suppression studies (page 5). *[No change in urine 17-OHCS levels with dexamethasone 8 mg/day.]*

4. The source of ACTH needs to be identified. A liver biopsy was performed showing cells compatible with adenocarcinoma. To follow up the hematochezia, a barium enema was ordered.

SEVERE WEAKNESS AND RECTAL BLEEDING   39

[A constricting nonocclusive lesion in the descending colon was found.] An exploratory laparotomy was performed. The colonic lesion was a moderately differentiated adenocarcinoma. Multiple metastatic nodules were noted in the omentum and liver.

5. Ideally, removal of the tumor would cure the syndrome, but that was not possible in this patient. In view of the widespread metastases, the surgeon chose not to perform bilateral adrenalectomy. Blockade of adrenalocorticoid synthesis often helps the hypokalemic alkalosis. Metyrapone (500 mg every 6 hours) was administered to this patient. Other medications such as aminogluthemide (0.5-1.5 mg/day), trilostane (120-240 mg/day), and ketoconazole (400-800 mg/day), alone or in combination, are often used.

PEARLS:

1. The clinical features of ectopic ACTH syndrome often differ from other causes of Cushing's syndrome. Ectopic ACTH syndrome is more common in males. Its clinical course is rapid (< 6 months' duration) and is associated with profound weakness. Often, hypokalemia and extreme hyperpigmentation provide helpful clues to aid in the diagnosis.

2. Up to 50% of patients with hypercortisolism due to ectopic ACTH syndrome have oat cell carcinoma of the lung. Carcinoid tumors are next most frequent (bronchial carcinoids predominate). Other tumors that may cause the syndrome are thymomas, pancreatic islet cell tumors, medullary thyroid carcinoma, and pheochromocytoma.

3. Many other tumors rarely cause ectopic ACTH syndrome. These include squamous carcinomas of lung, larynx, and

40 CASE STUDIES IN ENDOCRINOLOGY

cervix; adenocarcinomas of the colon (as in this case), lung, breast, ovary, ileum, and prostate; and melanoma and salivary gland tumors.

4. Not only can tumors make ACTH, but several cases of tumor production of corticotropin-releasing factor (CRF) have been reported. CRF causes the pituitary to secrete abundant amounts of ACTH and thus mimics ectopic ACTH syndrome.

5. Bilateral adrenalectomy is beneficial in patients with slow growing malignancies or with a tumor of unknown source secreting ACTH.

PITFALLS:

1. The clinical syndrome of ectopic ACTH varies dramatically. Typically, the patient with a known malignancy presents with profound weakness and metabolic hypokalemic alkalosis. Signs of chronic hypercortisolism are absent. However, there are indolent variants (particularly the bronchial carcinoid) that mimic Cushing's disease (pituitary-dependent adrenal hyperplasia) in nearly every aspect, including biochemical studies (suppression to high dose dexamethasone and exaggerated 17-OHCS response to metyrapone—see pages 270-271).

2. Some patients have had unsuccessful transsphenoidal surgery for Cushing's disease and later a lung lesion is found on chest X-ray or CT.

3. When the biochemical studies for Cushing's disease are not conclusive, order chest CT even when the chest X-ray is "normal." CT of the chest and abdomen appears to be more

accurate than venous sampling of ACTH to localize ACTH-secreting tumors.

REFERENCES

Belsky JL, Cuello B, Swanson LW, et al: Cushing's syndrome due to ectopic production of corticotropin-releasing factor. J Clin Endocrinol Metab 60:496, 1985.

Carey RM, Varna SK, Drake CR Jr, et al: Ectopic secretion of corticotropin-releasing factor as a cause of Cushing's syndrome. N Engl J Med 311:13, 1984.

Davies CJ, Joplin GR, Welbourn RB: Surgical management of the ectopic ACTH syndrome. Ann Surg 196:246, 1982.

Findling JW, Tyrrell JB: Occult ectopic secretion of corticotropin. Arch Intern Med 146:929, 1986.

Jex RK, van Heerden JA, Carpenter PC, Grant CS: Ectopic ACTH syndrome: diagnostic and therapeutic aspects. Am J Surg 149:276, 1985.

Liddle GW, Givens JR, Nicholson WE, Island DP: The ectopic ACTH syndrome. Cancer Res 25:1056, 1965.

White FE, White FC, Drury PL, et al: Value of computed tomography on the abdomen and chest in investigation of Cushing's syndrome. Br Med J 284:771, 1982.

WEAKNESS AND HYPERPIGMENTATION

CASE 6: J.B., a 40-year-old carpenter, complained of fatigue and weakness. His fatigue began about 6 months earlier. He attributed the tiredness to heat and working 10 to 11 hours each day while framing houses during the midsummer. During the fall, however, the work load was lighter, yet he could just barely make it to the end of the day. He experienced light-headedness but never actually fainted. He often felt nauseated but never vomited. He found himself adding salt to almost every food, something he had never done before. He denied any weight loss, fever, chills, increased urine frequency, headache, diarrhea, palpitations, pain in any joints or muscles, or use of any medications. His wife noted that he had never lost his summer's tan and questioned whether his weight might have decreased a few pounds. Family history revealed that his mother had hypothyroidism, but no other members had any known endocrine disease.

On physical examination, his weight was 145 lb; height, 68 inches; BP while lying down was 110/70 with a pulse of 68/min; BP while standing was 95/60 with a pulse of 84/min without any symptoms. He was a pleasant, dark-complected white male. The skin showed generalized melanosis that was particularly uncommon during the winter at 40° latitude. The melanosis was accentuated over the sun-exposed areas, the scrotum and perineum, nipple areola, and in the skin creases. Several small hyperpigmented areas over the gingival and buccal mucosa were found. HEENT, chest, abdominal, and neurological exams were normal.

WEAKNESS AND HYPERPIGMENTATION   43

ENDOCRINE CLUE: Serum studies: Na, 134 mEq/l; K, 5.4 mEq/l; BUN, 32 mg/dl; and creatinine, 1.1 mg/dl.

QUESTIONS:

1. What is your working diagnosis, and what other possibilities are less likely?

2. What studies would you order to work up this patient?

3. What caused his problem?

4. How would you manage this patient?

44   CASE STUDIES IN ENDOCRINOLOGY

ANSWERS:

1. Primary adrenal insufficiency (Addison's disease) seems most likely. The hyperpigmentation is the real tip-off. Other problems associated with increased pigmentation such as hyperthyroidism, severe chronic illness, Cushing's syndrome (low grade ectopic ACTH syndrome), hemochromatosis, or use of phenothiazine drugs seem unlikely. His postural hypotension, mild hyponatremia, and hyperkalemia suggest mineralo-corticoid deficiency. The increased serum BUN/creatinine ratio reflects the prerenal azotemia of salt wasting and volume contraction.

2. Low AM serum cortisol and elevated plasma ACTH levels are the diagnostic laboratory findings in Addison's disease. So order an AM cortisol and ACTH level. *[These values return: serum cortisol, 2 μg/dl; plasma ACTH, 900 pg/ml (normal, 20-80 pg/ml).]* In this patient, who has a classic presentation with low serum cortisol and high plasma ACTH values, further studies are not necessary. In practice, the ACTH level often returns much later, so that this critical information is not readily available to you. You need to be sure of the diagnosis of adrenal insufficiency because you are committing the patient to lifelong steroid replacement. Thus, one usually administers ACTH and looks for a failure of the serum cortisol and urine 17-OHCS or free cortisol (UC) to rise. A short ACTH test (though a great outpatient screening study) would be inferior to a more prolonged inpatient test of adrenal stimulation with ACTH to establish the diagnosis of adrenal insufficiency. Order a 24-hour urine as baseline for 17-OHCS and/or UC. Administer synthetic 1-24 ACTH (cosyntropin) 0.25 mg in 500 ml of saline over an 8-hour infusion (8 AM to 4 PM) on three consecutive days with concomitant 24-hour urine collections for 17-OHCS and/or UC determinations. Patients with primary adrenal insufficiency have no rise in the 17-OHCS or UC, whereas patients with secondary adrenal

WEAKNESS AND HYPERPIGMENTATION   45

insufficiency have a subnormal rise on the first day (less than three times basal 17-OHCS) and increase to three times the baseline by the third day. A shorter method using a 48-hour continuous infusion (cosyntropin 0.25 mg in 500 ml of normal saline every 12 hours) is equally valid (normal response: urine 17-OHCS > 27 mg for first 24 hours; > 47 mg in the second 24 hours).

3. At least 80% of Addisonian patients are presumed to have adrenal atrophy on an autoimmune basis. Lymphocytic infiltration may make the adrenals appear normal in size on CT scan. Antiadrenal antibodies are often present in serum. Granulomatous diseases (tuberculosis, histoplasmosis, and sarcoidosis) and rarely infiltrative diseases (amyloid, lymphoma, hemochromatosis, and metastatic carcinoma) are possible but not likely in this patient. Neither is hemorrhage into the adrenals that is seen in patients taking anticoagulant medication. The patient's age, normal neurological exam, and a negative family history make adrenoleukodystrophy very unlikely.

4. This patient requires maintenance steroid therapy. Hydrocortisone (cortisol) 20-30 mg/day is usually given twice a day, 10-20 mg at 7-8 AM and 10 mg at 4-6 PM. An occasional patient may need 10 mg three times a day. Hydrocortisone is rapidly absorbed from the gut and serum levels of cortisol peak after about 1 hour. Cortisone acetate may also be used for replacement. The dose is 25-37.5 mg/day given as 12.5-25 mg each AM and 12.5 mg each PM (identical to the hydrocortisone schedule). Cortisone acetate costs more than hydrocortisone. Since the half-life of cortisol is 60-90 minutes, the serum cortisol falls to < 3 µg/dl in the Addisonian patient 6-7 hours after ingesting replacement doses. To evaluate whether replacement dosage is adequate, the clinician must assess the patient for signs and symptoms of inadequate or excessive steroid

46 CASE STUDIES IN ENDOCRINOLOGY

replacement. Measurement of urine free cortisol in patients on replacement therapy is helpful in assuring proper doses of either hydrocortisone or cortisone acetate. Most patients with primary adrenal insufficiency need mineralocorticoid supplementation, although some patients will do well on glucocorticoid therapy alone with liberal salt intake. Fludrocortisone is the mineralocorticoid preparation of choice because it is potent, has prolonged activity, and is less expensive than aldosterone or deoxycorticosterone. The dose of fludrocortisone is 0.05-0.1 mg given as a single dose once a day or every other day as needed.

During times of stress (acute illness, fever, surgery, etc.), the patient should triple his daily maintenance dose of glucocorticoid and drop back to maintenance doses when the stress passes. Patients requiring surgery need continuous intravenous infusion of hydrocortisone sodium succinate (100 mg every 8 hours). Teaching Addisonian patients what to do in times of illness is extremely important. Patients should have intramuscular glucocorticoids available for emergencies and when they are unable to take medications by mouth. Make sure they wear a medallion identifying their diagnosis and steroid dependence.

PEARLS:

1. The grayish-brown color of hemochromatosis might be confused with the melanosis of adrenal insufficiency, but hemochromatosis is not likely to involve the mucous membranes (unlike patients with adrenal insufficiency in whom buccal mucosa is typical affected).

WEAKNESS AND HYPERPIGMENTATION   47

2. Stone-hard pinna caused by calcified auricular cartilage, though not diagnostic, provide a helpful clue in thinking about adrenal insufficiency.

3. Other endocrine diseases are often associated with adrenal insufficiency. Addisonian patients with idiopathic adrenal insufficiency need to be observed for the development of pernicious anemia, hypothyroidism (Schmidt's syndrome), diabetes mellitus, or hypoparathyroidism.

4. Hypercalcemia is found in up to 6% of patients with adrenal insufficiency. The cause of the hypercalcemia is poorly understood; however, correction of the hypocortisolemia readily normalizes the serum calcium.

5. Eosinophilia is relatively frequent and hypoglycemia is relatively infrequent in Addison's disease.

PITFALLS:

1. Not all patients with chronic adrenal insufficiency are hyperpigmented. Since about 8% of Addisonian patients do not have the classical hyperpigmentation, one must rely on a high index of suspicion to make the diagnosis (weakness and weight loss are nearly always present).

2. The patient with tuberculosis may develop weakness, hypotension, and weight loss while being treated with rifampin. Rifampin may unmask adrenal insufficiency or precipitate an Addisonian crisis by accelerating hepatic metabolism of cortisol. Hypoadrenal patients taking rifampin need two to three times the amount of replacement glucocorticoid to avoid hypoadrenalism.

48   CASE STUDIES IN ENDOCRINOLOGY

3. Failure to educate the Addisonian patient regarding the importance of steroid replacement, supplementation in times of stress, and wearing of proper identification leads to frequent complications, including death.

REFERENCES

Barnett AH, Espiner EA, Donald RA: Patients presenting with Addison's disease need not be pigmented. Postgrad Med J 58:690, 1982.

Burch WM: Urine-free cortisol determination: a useful tool in the management of chronic hypoadrenal states. JAMA 247:2002, 1982.

Kyriazopoulou V, Parparousi O, Vagenakis AG: Rifampicin-induced adrenal crisis in addisonian patients receiving corticosteroid replacement therapy. J Clin Endocrinol Metab 59:1204, 1984.

Nelson D: Diagnosis and treatment of Addison's disease. In DeGroot LJ, et al (eds): Endocrinology. New York, Grune & Stratton, 1979, pp 1193-1201.

Nerup J: Addison's disease-clinical studies. A report of 108 cases. Acta Endocrinol 76:127, 1974.

ANTERIOR NECK MASSES

CASE 7: S.W., a 29-year-old cook, came to the outpatient clinic stating that her gynecologist found a neck mass during her annual physical exam. She admitted to noticing some fullness in this area for a couple of years but could not precisely date its onset. There was no history of neck pain or tenderness, fever, menstrual irregularity, hoarseness, radiation exposure, or anxiety (except over the presence of this "mass"). She had gained 30 lb over the last year. She denied any use of medications or any family history of thyroid disease.

This woman was overweight (167 lb; height, 64 inches). The obesity was generalized and not limited to the trunk. On inspection, there was a prominent fullness in the mid-anterior neck located below the hyoid area. On palpation, the mass was symmetrical and had ill-defined margins measuring 7 cm in width and 5 cm in height. Its consistency was supple without any areas of firmness or discreet nodularity. It did not move when the patient swallowed water. No other neck masses were palpable. The remainder of the examination was normal.

ENDOCRINE CLUE: Technetium-99m pertechnetate scan of the anterior neck revealed the following:

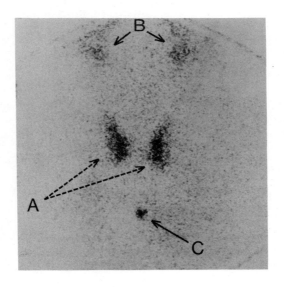

ANTERIOR NECK MASS   51

QUESTIONS:

1. What is the differential diagnosis in this patient?

2. What studies would help define her diagnosis?

3. What treatment would you recommend for the most likely diagnosis?

52   CASE STUDIES IN ENDOCRINOLOGY

ANSWERS:

1. The differential of midline anterior neck masses includes thyromegaly, thyroglossal duct remnant, laryngeal lesions, and pseudogoiter. In this patient, thyromegaly of the nontoxic diffuse variety (simple goiter) or thyroid cyst is possible, though unlikely. The absence of firmness and nodularity argues against Hashimoto's thyroiditis, anaplastic cancer, or infiltrative lymphoma. An enlarged pyramidal lobe of the thyroid is usually associated with enlargement of the lateral lobes of the thyroid as well. A thyroglossal duct cyst could present in this manner, but usually the margins are better delineated and the remnant duct cyst usually smaller than what is described in this patient.

Pseudogoiter exists when any fullness in the neck leads the physician to make a diagnosis of goiter when, in fact, an enlarged thyroid is not present. In most cases, pseudogoiter represents prominent adipose tissue (fat pad goiter). When a normal sized thyroid gland is located more superiorly in the neck, it becomes more prominent, leading a diagnosis of pseudogoiter secondary to a "high lying thyroid." Rarely, a delphian node (located between the hyoid bone and thyroid cartilage), dermoid cyst, parathyroid cyst, laryngeal lesion, or lipoma might present as pseudogoiter.

2. This patient's technetium scan identified normal functioning thyroid tissue that was not enlarged on imaging (see CLUE; marked **A**). The thyroid was in a normal position. The submaxillary salivary glands also concentrate technetium (marked **B**). A marker was placed on the suprasternal notch (**C**). Furthermore, the mass did not move on swallowing: a tip-off that it was not part of the thyroid or larynx. Physicians with experience in palpating neck masses may not order any further studies (assuming the diagnosis is pseudogoiter secondary to prominent adipose tissue). CT scan and secondary to prominent adipose tissue). CT scan and ultrasonography of the neck are quite useful in evaluating neck masses, but are not necessary for this patient.

3. In absence of any thyroid abnormality, a <u>diagnosis of pseudogoiter secondary to increased adipose tissue (fat pad goiter)</u> was made. The patient was reassured of no thyroid abnormality and advised to lose weight.

PEARLS:

1. <u>Always examine the thyroid gland while the patient is seated or standing.</u> Frequently, thyromegaly and thyroid nodules are not appreciated while the patient is lying supine.

2. An important part of the thyroid examination is to have the patient swallow. <u>Providing a cup of water will aid swallowing.</u>

3. An anterior neck mass that suddenly appears (within a day or so) suggests hemorrhage into a previously unrecognized thyroid cyst or thyroid adenoma.

4. A diffusely enlarged thyroid that is firm and hard suggests an infiltrative process such as Hashimoto's thyroiditis, lymphoma, anaplastic thyroid carcinoma, or Reidel's struma.

5. Cystic masses in the lateral anterior neck are most likely to be thyroid cysts. Branchial cleft cysts, cystic hygromas, or rarely parathyroid cysts should also be considered. CT scan is helpful in determining location, size, extent, and character of these neck masses.

54 CASE STUDIES IN ENDOCRINOLOGY

6. Levels of thyroglobulin are extremely high in fluid from thyroid cysts and are low in fluid from other neck cysts (e.g., parathyroid, dermoid, or branchial cleft cysts).

7. This page lists a helpful algorithm in evaluating neck masses (adapted from Linfors and Neelon).

NECK MASSES

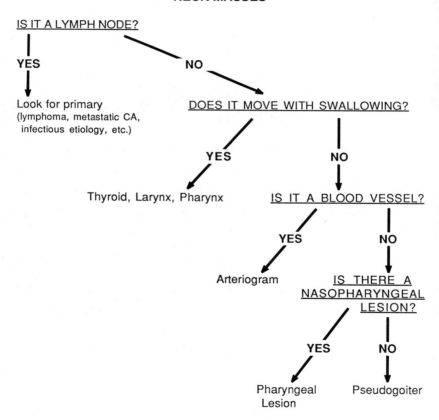

ANTERIOR NECK MASS   55

8. A <u>retroclavicular goiter</u> may produce respiratory distress and facial suffusion after neck flexion or elevation of the arms. These maneuvers cause thoracic inlet obstruction by the retroclavicular goiter and have been likened to the "pushing a cork" (goiter) further into "the bottle of the neck" (thoracic inlet). Pemberton described this sign (raising arms vertically above the head immediately adjacent to the face causes inspiratory stridor and facial plethora).

PITFALLS:

1. The thyroid gland is attached to the underlying tracheal cartilage. <u>Upon deglutition, the thyroid gland should move superiorly.</u> Failure of the mass to move should make you question whether the mass or nodule is intrinsic to the thyroid (as in this patient).

2. <u>Do not forget to transilluminate any neck masses.</u>

3. <u>Pseudogoiter</u> secondary to a <u>high lying thyroid</u> may be diagnosed when an experienced clinician palpates the thyroid to be normal in size or when the image on radionuclide scan is not enlarged and the anterior view demonstrates the midpoint of the isthmus lying more than 60% of the way from the suprasternal notch to the superior notch of the thyroid cartilage.

4. <u>Cervical lordosis</u> leading to swan-like configuration of the neck can produce pseudogoiter. Asking the patient to straighten his or her neck ameliorates the "goiter." This cause of pseudogoiter has been called <u>Modigliani syndrome</u> (after the long and exaggerated curved neck that distinguished the style of the artist Modigliani).

56 CASE STUDIES IN ENDOCRINOLOGY

5. Although thyroglossal duct cysts may have a benign course, surgical extirpation is indicated. These masses are often cosmetically unacceptable, have the potential for infection, and rarely harbor a carcinoma (over 100 cases of thyroid carcinoma have been reported within thyroglossal duct remnants).

6. In Cushing's syndrome, a soft, nontender fatty mass may form in the suprasternal notch. This should not be confused with thyromegaly.

REFERENCES

Blum M, Biller BJ, Bergman DA: The thyroid cork. Obstruction of the thoracic inlet due to retroclavicular goiter. JAMA 227:189, 1974.

Gwinup G, Morton ME: The high lying thyroid: a cause of pseudogoiter. J Clin Endocrinol Metab 40:37, 1975.

Linfors EW, Neelon FA: Neck masses: illustration of a logical approach. NC Med J 46:574, 1985.

LiVolsi VA, Perzin KH, Savetsky L: Carcinoma arising in median ectopic thyroid (including thyroglossal duct tissue). Cancer 34:1303, 1974.

Mercer RD: Pseudo-goiter: the Modigliani syndrome. Cleve Clin Q 42:319,1975.

NERVOUS PATIENT WITH ABNORMAL THYROID STUDIES

CASE 8: K.G., a 23-year-old textile employee, presented for an evaluation of nervousness. For the last 3 months she had had difficulty performing her job. She was employed in a textile mill as a doffer (removing spools of yarn from a spinning machine). Her productivity had decreased such that she was concerned about being laid off. When questioned about why she was doing poorly she replied, "I don't like my job or boss." She denied any heat or cold intolerance, weight loss, or change in her bowel habits. She had been diagnosed 2 years ago as having irritable bowel syndrome. She was married and had two children (ages 1 and 3). Her mother had a subtotal thyroidectomy for Graves' disease at the age 34.

She weighed 110 lb; pulse, 95/min; height, 62 inches. Her mental status and neurological exams were normal. HEENT exam revealed no proptosis, lid lag, or stare. Careful inspection and palpation of the neck identified no goiter or thyroid nodules. Chest and abdomen examinations were normal. The hands showed bitten fingernails without onycholysis.

ENDOCRINE CLUE: Serum thyroxine (T4-RIA) was 15.6 µg/dl (normal, 5-12). T3 uptake (T3U) was 34% (normal, 35-45). T3(RIA) was 210 ng/dl (normal, 90-190).

QUESTIONS:

1. What pertinent questions do you need ask the patient?

2. When the answers to Question #1 are known , can this woman be diagnosed as hyperthyroid? If she is hyperthyroid, what further studies are needed? If she is not hyperthyroid, why are the studies abnormal?

3. Would you recommend treatment?

58   CASE STUDIES IN ENDOCRINOLOGY

ANSWERS:

1. You need to know her menstrual history. <u>Is she pregnant</u>? *[No.]* <u>Are her menses regular and cyclic</u>? *[Yes.]* If she is using contraception, what form?   <u>Is she taking an oral contraceptive</u>? *[Yes.]* <u>What social and interpersonal problems might also contribute to her symptoms</u>? Is she a single parent trying to support children? Is there family strife?

2. <u>No</u>. This woman does not suffer from hyperthyroidism. Hyperthyroxinemia does not necessarily mean hyperthyroidism (a clinical diagnosis that results from the effects of excessive T4 and T3 levels). Her increased T4 level relates to an estrogen effect. Pregnancy and taking oral contraceptives raise thyroid binding globulin (TBG) levels. Since T4 and T3 circulate bound to TBG, the serum levels of T4 and T3 are increased. <u>The T3U value helps immensely in this case</u>. This patient's T3U level was below normal, leading to the conclusion that her TBG level was raised (see Pearl #1). In addition, her free thyroid index was normal (see Pearl #4). If her serum free T4 (FT4) were measured, the FT4 would be normal, as would her TSH response to thyrotropin-releasing hormone (see page 256).

3. <u>Avoid treatment with antithyroid drugs</u>. Explain that her thyroid studies are normal for a patient taking oral contraceptives. Reassurance, support, and counseling are appropriate avenues of therapy for her "nervousness."

PEARLS:

1. T3U measures indirectly the number of unoccupied protein binding sites for T4 and T3 in serum. The test gets its name from the radiolabeled T3 which is used in the in vitro assay.

NERVOUS PATIENT WITH ABNORMAL THYROID STUDIES 59

Radiolabeled T3 is added to the patient's serum and competes for binding sites on TBG. A resin or some other inert material is then added to adsorb any unbound radiolabeled T3. If TBG is increased, then the amount of radiolabeled T3 available for adsorption to the resin is less. The radioactivity of the resin is counted and expressed as percent of total counts added to the assay tube.

2. Radiolabeled T3 is used in the T3U assay instead of T4 because the assay time is shorter (T3 binding to TBG equilibrates faster than T4 binding). The normal range of values for T3U depends on the particular type of resin used, which means various laboratories have different normal ranges for T3U.

3. Here is a table that helps in interpreting T3U results.

Serum T3U -- Low	Serum T3U -- High
Increased TBG	*Decreased TBG*
Hyperestrogenic states	Androgen therapy
Estrogen therapy	Severe hypoproteinemia
Pregnancy	Major illness
Hydatidiform mole	
Estrogen-producing tumor	
Acute hepatitis	Chronic liver disease
Acute intermittent porphyria	Glucocorticoid excess
Hereditary TBG increase	Hereditary TBG deficiency
Myeloma	Acromegaly
Hypothyroidism	Hyperthyroidism
Drugs	
Perphenazine	Drugs that Bind to TBG
Methadone	Aspirin (high doses)
Heroin	Phenytoin
	Clofibrate
	Heparin

60   CASE STUDIES IN ENDOCRINOLOGY

4. Getting serum thyroxine levels alone without some estimate of TBG can cause much confusion. Measurement of T4 and T3U allows one to calculate a value called the free thyroid index (FTI). The FTI is an attempt to normalize discordant serum T4 and T3U values and is the product of the T4(RIA) multiplied by the T3U. This calculated number (FTI) correlates well with the levels of free T4.

5. Familial dysalbuminemic hyperthyroxinemia, an increasing recognized cause of increased serum T4, is caused by binding of T4 to an altered albumin which has great affinity for T4. A tip-off to this diagnosis is a symptom-free patient who has elevated serum T4 and normal serum T3U values.

6. Extremely ill patients and some psychiatric patients may have increased T4(RIA) levels due to decreased peripheral conversion of T4 to T3 (see page 268). The enzyme that normally removes the 5'-iodine from T4 to make T3 has decreased activity. However, deiodination of the 5-position continues leading to the formation of reverse T3. Thus, these patients have elevated levels of reverse T3. Although reverse T3 has no biological activity, it has been used as a marker in euthyroid sick patients. Whenever the sickness resolves, T4 levels and reverse T3 levels return to normal.

PITFALLS:

1. Be very careful in calling someone thyrotoxic in the absence of thyromegaly. Three to five percent of Graves' patients do not have a goiter. Though an enlarged thyroid gland need not be present in hyperthyroid patients, one ought to think twice before making a diagnosis of hyperthyroidism in the absence of thyromegaly. Two thyrotoxic conditions may not have an

NERVOUS PATIENT WITH ABNORMAL THYROID STUDIES 61

associated goiter: <u>painless thyroiditis</u> and <u>thyrotoxicosis factitia</u>.

2. <u>Remember that the T3U has nothing to do with the serum levels of T3.</u>

3. Serum T3 levels must be interpreted with the same caution as T4 levels (i.e., estrogens increase TBG levels, and since T3 circulates bound to TBG, serum T3 levels are also elevated).

4. More than one patient with presumed thyrotoxicosis has been treated definitively with radioactive iodine for hyperthyroxinemia. These patients include those with estrogen-induced increase in TBG, hereditary increase in TBG, and familial dysalbuminemic hyperthyroxinemia.

REFERENCES

Hershman JM: Use of thyrotropin-releasing hormone in clinical medicine. <u>Med Clin North Am</u> 62:313, 1978.

Ingbar SH: The thyroid gland. In Wilson JD, Foster DW (eds): <u>Textbook of Endocrinology</u>, ed. 7. Philadelphia, W.B. Saunders, 1985, pp 682-815.

Ruiz M, Rajatanavin R, Young RA, et al: Familial dysalbuminemic hyperthyroxinemia: a syndrome that can be confused with thyrotoxicosis. <u>N Engl J Med</u> 306:635, 1982.

Spaulding SW, Utiger RD: The thyroid: physiology, hyperthyroidism, hypothyroidism, and the painful thyroid. In Felig P, Baxter JD, Broadus AE, Frohman LA (eds): <u>Endocrinology and Metabolism</u>. New York, McGraw-Hill, 1981, pp 281-350.

THYROID NODULE

CASE 9: C.C., a 27-year-old legal secretary, came for her annual examination. She was entirely asymptomatic. Her prior health had been excellent. She delivered two healthy infants 2 and 4 years ago. Review of systems was normal: no change in weight, regular menses, no palpitations, and no history of prior neck or ear pain. She used a diaphragm for contraception. No history of head or neck irradiation was elicited. The family history was negative for any endocrine disease.

She weighed 134 lb; height, 65 inches; BP, 125/75; pulse, 75/min. The physical examination was normal except for a palpable asymmetrical mass (2 x 3 cm) located in the left anterior neck. The mass had smooth, well-defined margins, was moderately firm but not tender, did not transilluminate light, and moved when she swallowed. No other neck or supraclavicular masses were palpated.

ENDOCRINE CLUE: Routine laboratory studies were normal, including T4(RIA), 10.1 µg/dl (normal, 5-12); T3U, 38% (normal, 35-45); and serum calcium, 8.9 mg/dl.

THYROID NODULE   63

QUESTIONS:

1. What is the differential diagnosis for the solitary thyroid nodule?

2. What factors increase the risk for this nodule to be cancerous? What specific comments might you make about these factors?

3. Should this patient have a radionuclide thyroid scan?

4. What would you recommend next?

5. Given the findings noted in Question #4, what is the diagnosis?

6. What factors affect the prognosis of this disorder?

7. What is the treatment and follow-up for this problem?

64   CASE STUDIES IN ENDOCRINOLOGY

ANSWERS:

1. The possible diagnoses for solitary thyroid nodule are numerous. In this patient the diagnosis might be listed as follows (probability in decreasing order): <u>colloid nodule</u>; <u>thyroid cyst</u>; <u>benign adenoma</u>; <u>malignant tumor</u> (intrinsic lesions include papillary adenocarcinoma, follicular adenocarcinoma, medullary carcinoma, teratoma, and undifferentiated carcinoma, and extrinsic lesions include metastatic tumor, lymphoma, sarcoma, and squamous cell epidermoid carcinoma); <u>multinodular goiter</u> (even though only one nodule is palpable); and <u>miscellaneous disorders</u> such as focal thyroiditis and granulomatous disease (sarcoidosis, fungus).

2. The risk factors are: <u>age</u>; <u>sex</u>; <u>history of neck irradiation</u>; <u>family history of thyroid carcinoma</u>; and certain <u>physical characteristics of the thyroid itself</u>.

Age: Thyroid nodules are rare in children but about half of them are malignant. There is often a history of radiation exposure. Therefore, nodules found in patients under 16 years of age should be excised.

Sex: Thyroid nodules are five times more common in females than males. Thyroid cancer is also more frequent in females but only by a factor of two. Therefore, there is a greater risk of cancer for a male with a thyroid nodule than for a female.

History of irradiation: Irradiation of the head and neck (50-700 rads) is associated with an increased risk of thyroid cancer. The period of latency ranges from 5-35 years with the average around 20 years postexposure. Nodules should be removed in patients with this history.

History of familial thyroid carcinoma: Medullary thyroid carcinoma (sometimes associated with hyperparathyroidism and pheochromocytoma as multiple endocrine adenomatosis type II) is

THYROID NODULE   65

often familial. A family history for these possibilities should be sought.

Physical characteristics of the thyroid gland: The single nodule is much more likely to be malignant than the multinodular gland. The recent onset of a rapidly enlarging, firm neck mass (especially with associated hoarseness) is suggestive of infiltrative malignant disease. A thyroid mass presenting as a single palpable nodule (or as part of a multinodular gland) that is very firm, irregular, or adherent to overlying muscle generally needs surgical excision. Finally, carcinomatous thyroid cells do not trap radionuclides as well as normal thyroid cells, leading to a hypofunctioning or "cold" area on the thyroid scintiscan.

3. If a qualified cytopathologist is available to interpret fine needle aspiration biopsy, then thyroid scanning can be avoided. Most "cold" nodules are not malignant, and thus hypofunction of the nodule is not itself very helpful in making the decision to recommend surgery.

4. Although certain factors help to select high risk patients, only examination of tissue from the nodule is definite. In this regard fine needle aspiration helps immensely in the diagnosis and management of the solitary thyroid nodule. Surgical removal of all the high risk nodules leads to many patients having surgery for benign disease. Fine needle aspiration of these nodules offers a safe, rational approach to managing the thyroid nodule. The author uses the following technique of needle aspiration since small nodules can be well localized and fixed between the fingers to allow adequate sampling of thyroid tissue.

Thyroid masses are best palpated with the patient sitting or standing. The physician stands behind the patient, who sits upright in a chair. The area over the nodule is prepared with a local antiseptic. No local anesthetic is used. The nodule is fixed between the index and third finger. Having the patient swallow water will help center the nodule between these fingers, as demonstrated in Figure **A** (below). A 20-21 gauge needle is affixed to a plastic connecting tube which is attached to a 20-30 ml syringe. The hub of the needle is held between the thumb and index finger of the other hand (Fig. **B**). The needle is quickly inserted into the center of the mass. An assistant aspirates the obturator of the syringe to the 10-15 ml mark (Fig. **C**).

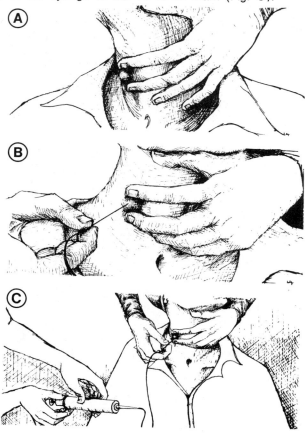

Method of Fine Needle Aspiration Biopsy: (**A**) The patient is seated in a chair and the nodule is localized. (**B**) Needle is inserted into the nodule. (**C**) An assistant aspirates the syringe.

THYROID NODULE 67

If fluid is obtained, the nodule can be massaged as the fluid is being aspirated. Any fluid is sent for cytology in a heparinized tube on ice. If no fluid is obtained, the tube is disconnected from the syringe, and then the needle removed from the nodule. Any scant material is forced by air onto a glass slide and fixed as any other cytological material (e.g., 70% ethanol). Multiple passes can be made to assure adequacy of the sample. The needle may be washed free of cells with normal saline into a heparinized tube and sent to the cytopathology laboratory on ice. There the cells can be washed with increasing concentrations of ethanol, which lyses red blood cells, filtered through a Millipore filter, and then stained for interpretation by the cytopathologist.

The cytopathological findings for our patient are given below:

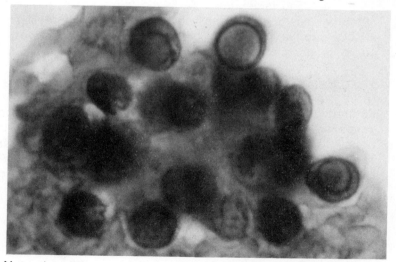

Note the different sizes of the nuclei, along with intranuclear inclusions (often called "Orphan Annie" nuclei). Also note the absence of colloid and inflammatory cells.

68   CASE STUDIES IN ENDOCRINOLOGY

5. The heterogeneity of nuclei and "Orphan Annie" cells are typical findings of papillary adenocarcinoma of the thyroid. Often, three-dimensional papillary fragments can be found.

6. Several factors affect the prognosis of thyroid carcinoma: cell type, age, and initial size of primary tumor. Histology does bear on the prognosis. Papillary and mixed papillary-follicular carcinoma behave similarly and have a benign course; follicular carcinoma is more aggressive. Anaplastic carcinoma has an extremely poor prognosis. The age of the patient at the time of diagnosis is a major prognostic feature. Young patients do well and seldom is there death from thyroid cancer below the age of 40 years. Papillary and mixed papillary-follicular cancers have a median onset age of 35 years, whereas follicular cancer occurs at a median age of 45 years. The larger the size of the initial tumor, the poorer the prognosis, but regional node metastasis of papillary or mixed papillary-follicular carcinoma does not adversely affect prognosis.

7. The management of thyroid carcinoma is controversial. The rarity, protracted course, and low mortality of well-differentiated carcinoma have made randomized treatment studies difficult to perform. It is generally agreed that the nodule should be removed and that thyroid suppressive therapy should be continued indefinitely. How much thyroid to remove (one lobe versus total thyroidectomy) and the best method to provide follow-up are unanswered variables.

Total thyroidectomy followed by 50-75 mCi of I-131 a month after surgery while the patient is hypothyroid (i.e., on no replacement thyroxine) will ablate any remaining functioning thyroid cells. Thyroid suppression with L-thyroxine is then instituted. Six months later after L-thyroxine is discontinued for at least a month, a total body I-131 scan is performed as follows: the patient is given 1-2 mCi of I-131 and then

THYROID NODULE 69

mCi of I-131 and then scintiscan is done 24 and 48 hours later. If the 6-month scan is negative, thyroxine suppression is reinstituted and the procedure is repeated in 12-18 months. If negative then, scans are performed no more frequently than every 5 years unless there is evidence of local recurrence. If functioning tissue is identified on any scan, then I-131 100-200 mCi is given, L-thyroxine is reinstituted, and the body scan is repeated 6 months later. This course is repeated as long as the scan is positive. Patients who are to receive > 30 mCi of I-131 are hospitalized in compliance with radiation safety standards. Patients are seen in yearly follow-up to assess the neck for recurrent nodules and for assurance that levels of serum T4 are maintained with L-thyroxine. This combination of total thyroidectomy, I-131 ablation, and thyroid suppression offers effective therapy.

PEARLS:

1. If there is clinical evidence of malignancy (e.g., a child with a single, firm thyroid nodule or history of radiation exposure), surgical removal is recommended. Otherwise, fine needle aspiration is routinely performed.

2. Some 15-20% of hypofunctioning or "cold" nodules are cysts and are best managed with needle aspiration.

3. <u>Any thyroid nodule that gradually enlarges on adequate thyroid suppression ought to be removed.</u>

4. On occasion, a solitary thyroid nodule may be caused by Hashimoto's thyroiditis. High titers of thyroid antimicrosomal antibodies should be expected.

70   CASE STUDIES IN ENDOCRINOLOGY

5. Thyroglobulin (produced by functioning thyroid cells but not C cells) is found in the serum in small amounts. Once the thyroid is ablated (e.g., by total thyroidectomy or by large doses of I-131), no serum thyroglobulin is detectable. The presence of any measurable serum thyroglobulin after total ablation suggests recurrence of the disease, since there should be no thyroid tissue remaining. The assay for serum thyroglobulin must be sensitive and specific to be useful.

PITFALLS:

1. If cytopathological interpretation of a fine needle aspirate is compatible with follicular adenoma, then surgery is advised since the cytopathologist cannot differentiate follicular adenoma from follicular adenocarcinoma. Often, the cytopathologist will call this finding "suspicious," which prompts surgical intervention.

2. The patient who is taking L-thyroxine for a thyroid nodule and experiences sudden enlargement of the nodule does not necessarily have cancer. Most likely, this represents hemorrhage into a adenoma or cyst. Aspiration will confirm this diagnosis.

3. A "nodule" that occupies the entire thyroid lobe may represent all that remains of normal thyroid tissue. The other lobe may be absent (thyroid hemiagenesis).

REFERENCES

Burch W: A method of fine-needle aspiration thyroid biopsy. Ann Intern Med 98:1023, 1983.

Burch WM: A method of aspirating thyroid cysts. Surg Gynecol Obstet 48:95, 1979.

Burrow GN: The thyroid: nodules and neoplasia. In Felig P, Baxter JD, Broadus AE, Frohman LA (eds): Endocrinology and Metabolism. New York, McGraw-Hill, 1981, pp 351-382.

DeGroot LJ, Larsen PR, Refetoff S, Stanbury JB. Thyroid neoplasia. The Thyroid and its Diseases, ed. 5. New York, John Wiley & Sons, 1984, pp 756-831.

Ingbar SH. The thyroid gland. In Wilson JD, Foster DW (eds): Textbook of Endocrinology, ed. 7. Philadelphia, W.B. Saunders Co., 1985, pp 682-815.

Mazzaferri EL, Young RL, Oertel JE, et al: Papillary thyroid carcinoma: the impact of therapy in 576 patients. Medicine 56:171, 1977.

van Herle AJ, Rich P, Ljung BME, et al: The thyroid nodule. Ann Intern Med 96:221, 1982.

UNILATERAL NECK MASS

CASE 10: R.H., a 75-year-old retired farmer, came to the gastrointestinal clinic for routine follow-up of a perforated prepyloric ulcer. That problem had resolved, but an anterior neck mass was noted. Baseline studies that included complete blood count (CBC), serum electrolytes, BUN, glucose, T4(RIA) and T3U were normal. A thyroid scan was obtained (see CLUE) and the patient was referred to the endocrine clinic. The patient was unaware of the mass until his physicians pointed it out to him. He denied any pain, dysphagia, hoarseness, insomnia, anxiety, fatigue, temperature intolerance, diarrhea, constipation, or any change in his skin. He had gained 10 lb over the last year. The patient had no past history of head or neck irradiation. His family history was negative for any endocrine disease.

On physical examination, BP was 150/88; pulse, regular at 64/min; height, 68 inches; weight, 195 lb. He appeared healthy with no lid lag, stare, or proptosis. A mass was apparent in the area of the right lobe of the thyroid. This mass palpated to be 2 cm wide x 3 cm high and moved on swallowing. The nodule was nontender, freely movable, and firm (but not rock hard) and had smooth margins. No cervical or axillary nodes were palpable. The remainder of the exam was entirely normal.

UNILATERAL NECK MASS 73

ENDOCRINE CLUE:

Technetium-99m pertechnetate scan of the anterior neck.

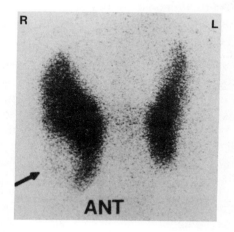

QUESTIONS:

1. What would you order next?

2. After you get the results of these studies, what is the diagnosis?

3. What other information and/or studies are indicated once you have established the diagnosis?

4. What is the treatment for this problem?

5. What factors affect the prognosis of this disorder?

74   CASE STUDIES IN ENDOCRINOLOGY

ANSWERS:

1. Because he is clinically euthyroid, confirmed by normal T4 and T3U, no further thyroid function studies are indicated. The thyroid scan demonstrates a hypofunctioning nodule in the right lobe of the thyroid. The possibilities include nonfunctioning thyroid adenoma, thyroid carcinoma, thyroid cyst, localized thyroiditis, lymphoma, or metastatic carcinoma. <u>The most efficacious study would be fine needle aspiration (FNA) biopsy of this nodule.</u> FNA provides tissue to define the underlying pathology and offers a means of treating cysts. Thyroid scanning costs more and gives less information. If this patient had been evaluated initially in the endocrine clinic, FNA biopsy would have been performed and thyroid scan would not have been ordered. The critical factor in needle aspiration is the availability of a cytopathologist who is expert in interpreting thyroid pathology. The results of FNA biopsy are shown below. The left panel demonstrates clumps of spindle-shaped cells with uniform nuclei. The right panel shows similar cells stained with an immunoperoxidase stain for calcitonin.

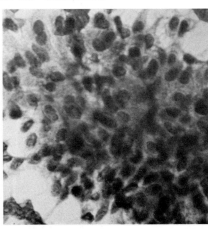 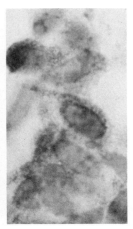

UNILATERAL NECK MASS   75

2. <u>Routine cytopathology of the FNA biopsy suggests medullary thyroid carcinoma.</u> The cells do not have a follicular or papillary pattern. The staining is positive for calcitonin, confirming the diagnosis of <u>medullary thyroid carcinoma</u> (MTC). Eighty percent of the cases of MTC present as sporadic MTC (similar to this patient). The age of patients with sporadic MTC averages in the mid-fifties. The diagnosis is frequently made following surgery for a solitary thyroid nodule. The remaining 20% of MTC cases are familial and are inherited as an autosomal dominant trait. There are three categories of familial MTC: **a**) <u>MEN IIa</u>-MTC, pheochromocytoma, hyperparathyroidism; **b**) <u>MEN IIb</u>-MTC, mucosal neuromas, pheochromocytoma, and marfanoid features; and **c**) <u>non-MEN familial MTC,</u> associated only with MTC. The average age of patients with familial MTC is in the twenties. Most likely, our patient has sporadic MTC (age 75 and negative family history).

3. Calcitonin secreted by the parafollicular or C cell is the biochemical marker for MTC. A <u>plasma calcitonin (CT) should be obtained</u>. *[CT level, 5000 pg/ml; normal levels are often nondectable or < 200 pg/ml.]* <u>Order a serum calcium</u> (to rule out hyperparathyroidism) and <u>a 24-hour urine for vanillylmandelic acid (VMA) or catecholamines</u> (to rule out pheochromocytoma). *[Ca, 9.8 mg/dl; VMA, 3.5 mg/gm creatinine.]* <u>Carcinoembryonic antigen (CEA)</u> was obtained in this patient. *[Negative.]* The possibility of familial MTC should be excluded. Baseline plasma calcitonin levels, if elevated are useful, but to detect the disease <u>early</u> in family members requires provocative testing. Since calcium and gastrin are potent secretagogues of calcitonin, plasma calcitonin levels are obtained at 0 time and at 2, 3.5, 5, and 7 minutes after calcium gluconate intravenously (2 mg of elemental Ca/kg over 1 minute) followed by a 10-second bolus of pentagastrin 0.5 µg/kg. A rise of > 300 pg/ml is diagnostic of C-cell hyperplasia or MTC. (Normal values of calcitonin vary

76 CASE STUDIES IN ENDOCRINOLOGY

depending on the assay. Each laboratory should establish its own reference levels.)

4. Surgery is the only effective treatment for MTC. Early detection of MTC in family members is possible using provocative testing and, with total thyroidectomy, represents the only way to cure this disease. Parathyroid reimplantation into forearm muscle usually prevents surgical hypoparathyroidism. Maintenance doses of T4 (1 µg/lb) are administrated postoperatively.

5. Several factors affect the prognosis of MTC. a) The type of MTC: MEN IIb-associated MTCs tend to be very aggressive (early metastases and infiltrating lesions) whereas non-MEN MTCs have a good prognosis. The biology of aggressiveness is: MEN IIb > MEN IIa > sporadic MTC > non-MEN MTC. b) The size of the primary mass correlates with prognosis (the larger the mass, the worse the outcome). c) The level of plasma calcitonin: Levels of calcitonin above 10,000 ng/ml are associated with high mortality. Lesser elevations of calcitonin are associated with higher survival rates. d) The degree of calcitonin-immunoperoxidase staining of the tumor: High levels of reactivity (> 75% staining) are associated with good prognosis. Low levels of staining predict poor outcome.

PEARLS:

1. MTC accounts for 4-10% of all thyroid carcinoma. MTC cells not only secrete calcitonin but may produce a host of bioactive products, including ACTH (causing Cushing's syndrome), beta-lipotropin, prostaglandins, serotonin, and CEA.

UNILATERAL NECK MASS   77

2. <u>The importance of early diagnosis of MEN-associated MTC cannot be overemphasized</u>. The only way to cure these clinically occult cases of MTC is to identify them early (using calcium and pentagastrin testing) and perform total thyroidectomy. Screening of family members every 6-12 months with provocative testing is strongly recommended.

3. Because familial MTC is usually bilateral and MTC tends to metastasize to central lymph nodes, total thyroidectomy and biopsy of paratracheal and upper mediastinal nodes are necessary.

4. The stimulated level of plasma calcitonin provoked by calcium and pentagastrin administration has prognostic significance. Patients with calcitonin levels < 1000 pg/mg have C-cell hyperplasia or microinvasive MTC. Surgery cures these patients (cure rate, 95%). If calcitonin levels are > 10,000 pg/ml, palpable disease is likely. There is a higher incidence of regional lymph node metastases, residual MTC postoperatively, distant metastases, and early death in these patients. In these subjects, the cure rate is about 40%.

5. Immunostaining of primary tumors has prognostic value. Patients with calcitonin-rich MTC (> 75% of cells stained for calcitonin) have a 5-year survival rate of 100% compared to 53% for patients whose tumor stains poorly for calcitonin (< 25% of cells stained for calcitonin). Calcitonin-rich metastases are compatible with prolonged survival, whereas calcitonin-poor metastases have poor survival.

6. CEA has been used as a prognostic indicator of disease. CEA, a fetal antigen, appears to be a marker for early epithelial differentiation, whereas calcitonin serves as a marker of terminal cell differentiation or maturity. CEA levels are generally higher in patients with metastatic disease.

78   CASE STUDIES IN ENDOCRINOLOGY

PITFALLS:

1. In patients with suspected MTC, get a 24-hour urine for catecholamines or VMA prior to surgical intervention in the neck. Remove the pheochromocytoma (often bilateral) before operating on the thyroid (and parathyroid glands).

2. Measurement of plasma calcitonin in every patient with a thyroid nodule is not practical or reasonable. If the clinical picture suggests MTC, then order a calcitonin level. The patient with thyroid nodule(s) and diarrhea, spells and hypertension (pheochromocytoma), hypercalcemia (hyperparathyroidism), or mucosal neuromas (MEN IIb) deserves a calcitonin determination.

3. Plasma calcitonin levels often remain elevated after thyroidectomy in absence of any overt metastases. CEA levels might be more helpful in follow-up. Rising CEA levels indicate a poor prognosis in the face of stable or decreasing calcitonin levels. CEA appears to be secreted by calcitonin-poor staining metastases which have virulent behavior.

REFERENCES

Kini SR, Miller JM, Hamburger JI, Smith MJ: Cytopathologic features of medullary carcinoma of the thyroid. Arch Pathol Lab Med 108:156, 1984.

Saad MF, Ordonez NG, Guido JJ, Samaan NA: The prognostic value of calcitonin immunostaining in medullary carcinoma of the thyroid. J Clin Endocrinol Metab 59:850, 1984.

Saad MF, Ordonez NG, Rashid RK, et al: Medullary carcinoma of thyroid. Medicine 63:319, 1984.

Wells SA Jr, Dilley WD, Farndon JA, et al: Early diagnosis and treatment of medullary thyroid carcinoma. Arch Intern Med 145:1248, 1984.

PRURITUS AND WEIGHT LOSS

CASE 11: D.G., a 26-year-old school teacher, presented complaining of itchy skin and of being excessively nervous and jittery. Her symptoms started about two months ago. She was "short-tempered," easily angered, and tremulous. About four weeks ago, pruritus developed over the anterior and posterior chest that was unassociated with a rash. Nothing seemed to help the itch. She lost 5 lb despite a voracious appetite, perspired much more than normal, and preferred a cool room with the thermostat set at 60-65°F. She denied any diarrhea, polyuria, cough, headache, medication use, or change in menses. Her mother had been treated for hyperthyroidism 15 years ago.

She could not seem to sit still during the examination. Her weight was 125 lb; height, 65 inches; pulse, 98/min; BP, 110/60. Her hands were red, warm, and moist. The CLUE shows her fingernails. HEENT: No exophthalmos or stare was observed. The thyroid was easily visible. On palpation the total thyroid width was 7 cm, with each lobe measuring 5 cm in height. The gland was moderately firm and symmetrically enlarged without any palpable nodules. A venous hum was heard at the base of the right lobe of the thyroid. The heart, lung, and abdominal exams were normal. A fine tremor of outstretched fingers, brisk deep tendon reflexes, and lid lag were noted.

80 CASE STUDIES IN ENDOCRINOLOGY

ENDOCRINE CLUE: Photograph of fingers.

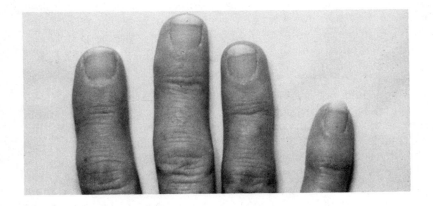

PRURITUS AND WEIGHT LOSS   81

QUESTIONS:

1. What is the diagnosis?

2. What are the possible causes of this disorder?

3. What is the most useful study to help you to diagnosis the etiology of the problem?

4. Why might the thyroid be called a "bystander" in this condition?

5. What therapies are available to manage this problem?

6. What treatment would you recommend to this patient? Why?

7. What should the patient expect after this treatment is administered?

82   CASE STUDIES IN ENDOCRINOLOGY

ANSWERS:

1. Hyperthyroidism (thyrotoxicosis). The history of weight loss, increased adrenergic symptoms, early onycholysis (see CLUE), and diffuse thyromegaly establish the diagnosis of hyperthyroidism. The onycholysis is subtle but definite. Typically, the third or fourth fingernail shows receding subungual margins that lead to loss of curvature (straightening) and then further regression (see page 263.).

2. Hyperthyroidism may be caused by increased secretion of thyroid hormones (T3 and T4) by overactive follicles (e.g., Graves' disease or iodine loading in susceptible patients) or by release of stored T3 and T4 (e.g., thyroiditis). Less likely causes include taking too much thyroid medication or trophoblastic disease.

3. Serum T4(RIA) and T3U levels should be high in all the conditions listed above. The 24 hour I-131 thyroidal uptake provides the most helpful information as to the etiology of the hyperthyroidism. In Graves' disease, the uptake is elevated. In thyroiditis, iodine loading, and surreptitious use of thyroid, the uptake is low. [This patient's 24-hour thyroidal uptake was 52%, making diffuse toxic goiter the diagnosis.]

4. Patients with diffuse toxic goiter or Graves' disease (hyperthyroidism with ophthalmopathy) have thyroid glands that are infiltrated with lymphocytes. These activated lymphocytes (Ia positive) produce immunoglobulins that bind to the thyroid-stimulating hormone (TSH) receptor. After binding of the IgG-TSH receptor complex, the thyroid follicle produces and secretes excessive amounts of T3 and T4. What triggers or activates this subset of lymphocytes is unknown. Furthermore, what causes them to cease immunoglobulin production is equally an enigma. The thyroid, though a

PRURITUS AND WEIGHT LOSS   83

bystander caught in an immunological war, contributes almost totally to the clinical syndrome of hyperthyroidism.

5. A method that treats the cause of this disorder would be the optimal therapy. At present, the best one can do is to control the hyperthyroidism with antithyroid drugs until the basic disease process undergoes spontaneous remission. Unfortunately, spontaneous remission occurs in only 20-30% of patients in the United States. Therefore, the clinician must decide on long-term antithyroid medication or on some form of ablative thyroid therapy such as radioactive iodine, or much less frequently, subtotal thyroidectomy.

6. I-131 therapy is the treatment of choice for most adults with Graves' disease. Patients who have failed with long-term thionamides (propylthiouracil or methimazole) are also treated with I-131. It is safe, inexpensive, effective, and convenient; pregnancy is the only absolute contraindication. Most patients are treated as outpatients. Younger patients may be treated while they are still hyperthyroid and covered with beta-adrenergic blockers. For this woman, one should prescribe propranolol 20-40 mg four times a day prior to the administration of I-131 and continue the propranolol until she is euthyroid. The dose of I-131 is generally 5-15 mCi. The lower dose is associated with lower incidence of hypothyroidism but a higher incidence of unresolved hyperthyroidism. High doses of I-131 reverse these incidences.

7. Within 6-12 weeks after I-131 treatment, the patient is generally euthyroid and propranolol is discontinued. If the patient is still hyperthyroid 6-12 months after I-131, a second treatment is necessary. The incidence of hypothyroidism that develops depends on treatment dose and ranges from 20 to 70%. Surveillance for hypothyroidism must continue for the life of the patient. Practically, it is

84   CASE STUDIES IN ENDOCRINOLOGY

easier to manage the patient if there is good ablation leading to hypothyroidism. This complication is acceptable since thyroid hormone replacement is easily managed with L-thyroxine 0.1-0.2 mg/day at a cost of $.06 or less per day. Good follow-up is necessary to treat hypothyroidism early or to detect the recurrence of hyperthyroidism.

PEARLS:

1. Elderly or especially ill, hyperthyroid patients are treated with thionamides until euthyroid, then the thionamide is discontinued for 4-7 days and I-131 is given. This reduces the amount of thyroid hormone released after radiation injury and avoids the cardiovascular effects that may occur with a sudden surge in the serum levels of thyroid hormones.

2. At present there are no reliable markers to define the population that will undergo spontaneous remission while on thionamide therapy.

3. Clinically there are two groups that respond well to long-term thionamide treatment: patients with small thyroid glands and those whose hyperthyroidism is of very recent onset.

4. The introduction of beta-adrenergic antagonists has had a major influence on the management of hyperthyroidism. Propranolol is the most commonly used blocker. Propranolol alleviates but does not totally resolve many of the symptoms of hyperthyroidism such as tachycardia, sweating, tremor, heat intolerance, and anxiety. The usual dose is 20-40 mg four times a day.

PRURITUS AND WEIGHT LOSS   85

5. Pruritus is not an uncommon manifestation of hyperthyroidism. The cause is unknown.

6. Hyperthyroid patients who surreptitiously take excessive thyroid medications (thyrotoxicosis factitia) have low I-131 uptake and do not have a goiter (unless it existed prior to thyroid administration).

PITFALLS:

1. Women may complain that their scalp hair falls out several weeks to months after treatment for thyrotoxicosis, when they are now euthyroid. Remind them that hair grows in cycles and stages, and that illness such as hyperthyroidism tends to put hairs into the same cycle. Thus, large amounts of hair may shed. This is not due to the I-131 treatment and may occur with any effective therapy for hyperthyroidism.

2. Patients who have thyrotoxicosis secondary to painless thyroiditis do not need thionamide treatment. Propranolol administration suffices in this self-limited disorder. If pain is a problem, then aspirin 650 mg four times a day may be prescribed.

3. Hypercalcemia in the thyrotoxic patient usually resolves as the hyperthyroidism ameliorates. Persistent hypercalcemia in the euthyroid patient requires evaluation.

REFERENCE

DeGroot LJ, Larsen PR, Refetoff S, Stanbury JB. Graves' disease and the manifestations of thyrotoxicosis. The Thyroid and its Diseases, ed. 5. New York, John Wiley & Sons, 1984, pp 341-398.

GOITER AND ATRIAL FIBRILLATION

CASE 12: T.N., a 68-year-old widow, was admitted for a fractured hip after she had slipped on an icy sidewalk. X-rays in the emergency room showed a subcapsular fracture of the left femoral head. After a preoperative ECG showed atrial fibrillation, a medicine consult was ordered.

Her health had been good. She had noted a fullness in the anterior neck for several years and had been told that this was a small goiter. She denied excessive nervousness or anxiety, only an occasional palpitation. Despite a good appetite, she had lost 4 lb over the last 8 weeks Recently she had a cough and took an expectorant. She denied any dysphagia, neck pain, dyspnea, polyuria, or chest pain. She had an uneventful menopause at the age of 54. She did not smoke or abuse alcohol. There was no family history of endocrine disease.

She was a thin, medium-frame female who was in no acute distress. BP was 125/70; brachial pulse, irregular at 104/min; heart rate, 135/min on rhythm strip; and temperature, 98.8°F. Other than the tachyarrhythmia, abnormal findings included an enlarged thyroid and a shortened left leg that was rotated laterally. The thyroid contained three distinct nodules (each 1-3 cm in diameter). The thyroid was estimated to be at least two times normal size (lying on a gurney made accurate assessment difficult). The skin was unexpectedly smooth and soft.

ENDOCRINE CLUE: The combination of atrial tachyarrhythmia and long-standing goiter should raise the possibility of thyrotoxicosis.

GOITER AND ATRIAL FIBRILLATION   87

QUESTIONS:

1. What studies would you order?

2. Why should you be concerned about her cough medication?

3. What is the most likely diagnosis?

4. How is this disorder different from Graves' disease or iodine-induced hyperthyroidism?

5. How would you manage this patient?

88 CASE STUDIES IN ENDOCRINOLOGY

ANSWERS:

1. <u>T4(RIA), T3U, FTI,</u> *[T4, 14 µg/dl; T3U, 46%; FTI, 7 (2.2-5.5)].* If the T4 were normal, then a <u>serum T3</u> should be obtained to rule out T3-thyrotoxicosis. A <u>thyroidal uptake and scan,</u> though not necessary to make the diagnosis of hyperthyroidism, helps identify the cause. *[The I-131 uptake was 27% (normal, 10-30%) and the scan showed areas of increased and decreased activity.]*

2. Some cough medications and decongestants contain iodine. The patient who has a goiter is subject to the <u>Jod-Basedow phenomenon,</u> that is, iodine-induced hyperthyroidism. The following table lists some iodine-containing products.

Iodine cough mixtures (SSKI, etc.)
Quadrinal
Combid
Floraquin
Betadine
Amiodarone
Entero-Vioform
Clioquinal
Benziodarone
Phospholine iodine eyedrops
X-ray contrast media
Kelp
<u>Vitamin pills</u>

[This woman's expectorant contained no iodine. If it had, then the first step in treatment would be discontinue this medication.]

3. <u>Toxic nodular goiter.</u> She had a nodular thyroid gland and elevated thyroid function studies. This patient was relatively asymptomatic from her hyperthyroidism. In fact, had she not had a fractured hip she would not have been seen. Whether

GOITER AND ATRIAL FIBRILLATION   89

her hyperthyroidism is truly <u>apathetic hyperthyroidism</u> or insidious onset of <u>toxic multinodular goiter</u> is difficult to discern. Apathetic hyperthyroidism is a thyrotoxic state characterized by fatigue, lethargy, listlessness, extreme weakness, and often congestive heart failure.

4. Toxic multinodular goiter (TNG), Graves' disease, and iodine-induced hyperthyroidism (Jod-Basedow phenomenon) are identical in many aspects, that is, similar symptoms and signs of thyrotoxicosis. However, the underlying pathology is different so that some clinical and laboratory features are characteristic for each disorder. <u>Age</u>, <u>onset of symptoms of hyperthyroidism</u>, <u>family history of thyroid disease</u>, <u>presence of goiter</u>, <u>exophthalmos</u>, <u>thyroidal uptake</u>, <u>thyroidal scan</u>, <u>associated autoimmune disease</u>, <u>thyroid microsomal antibodies</u>, and <u>spontaneous remission</u>. This table points to some of these features.

	Toxic Nodular Goiter	Graves' Disease	Iodine-Induced Hyperthyroidism
<u>Age of onset (yr)</u>	50-70	10-40	40-70
<u>Onset of symptoms</u>	Insidious	Insidious	Acute
<u>Family history</u>	Infrequent	Frequent	Rare
<u>Goiter</u>	100%	97%	75%
<u>Character of goiter</u>	Nodular	Diffuse	Variable (often multinodular)
<u>Exophthalmos</u>	Rare	Frequent	Rare
<u>Thyroidal uptake</u>	Usually elevated	Elevated	Decreased
<u>Thyroidal scan</u>	Areas of increased uptake	Diffuse	Unable to visualize and decreased uptake
<u>Associated autoimmune disease</u>	Rare	Frequent	Rare
<u>Thyroid microsomal antibodies</u>	Absent	Often present	Infrequent
<u>Spontaneous remission</u>	Rare	May occur	Usually resolves following iodine withdrawal

90 CASE STUDIES IN ENDOCRINOLOGY

5. There are several ways in which this patient who was relatively asymptomatic could be managed. First, <u>achieve euthyroidism with antithyroid medications</u>. *[Administer propylthiouracil 200-300 mg every 8 hours by mouth. Beta-adrenergic agents were not used.]* Second, after being made euthyroid <u>most patients with toxic multinodular goiter are treated with ablative I-131 therapy</u>. Thionamides are not prescribed for long-term therapy since spontaneous remissions rarely, if ever, occur. <u>Large doses of I-131 (30-50 mCi) are necessary to ablate the thyroid, and multiple doses are often necessary to control the hyperthyroidism</u>. *[The patient received 50 mCi of I-131.]* Surgery may be used, especially for large goiters producing obstructive symptoms.

PEARLS:

1. Thyrotoxicosis should be carefully excluded in any goitrous patient with tachycardia or congestive heart failure.

2. When the thyroidal uptake of radioactive iodine is low and the patient is hyperthyroid, consider iodine-induced thyrotoxicosis as well as thyroiditis. Taking iodine-containing medication may increase the iodine pool, so that tracer amounts of radiolabeled iodine will not be incorporated in same degree, leading to lower uptakes.

3. Toxic adenomatous goiter was first described by H.S. Plummer and thus is sometimes called Plummer's disease.

4. The causes of hyperthyroidism listed in decreasing are: **a)** Graves' disease, **b)** thyroiditis, **c)** toxic multinodular goiter, **d)** toxic thyroid adenoma, **e)** exogenous hyperthyroidism (iatrogenic, factitious, iodine-induced), **f)** excess TSH (trophoblastic tumors, pituitary tumor), and **g)** ectopic

GOITER AND ATRIAL FIBRILLATION 91

thyroxine production (struma ovarii and metastatic follicular thyroid carcinoma).

5. Apathetic thyrotoxic patients often mask their hyperthyroidism involving one system (e.g., cardiovascular with congestive heart failure, angina, or unresponsive tachydysrhythmias; gastrointestinal or occult malignancy with weight loss and anorexia, nausea, and abdominal pain; or neuromuscular with muscle weakness/myopathy or depression—"thyroid melancholia"). Elderly patients are particularly susceptible to this uncommon form of hyperthyroidism.

6. Iodine-induced thyrotoxicosis usually disappears within a few months after iodine is discontinued. These patients often become more symptomatic immediately after iodine is withdrawn. Normally, iodine inhibits thyroid hormone synthesis (acute Wolff-Chaikoff effect) and tends to block thyroid hormone release. Unleashing this blockade (by iodine discontinuation) promotes release of stored hormone making the patient more thyrotoxic.

PITFALLS:

1. <u>Avoid using iodine preparations if possible in any patient with multinodular goiter</u> since the risk of precipitating hyperthyroidism is high (up to 40-50%). The same preparations may also cause hypothyroidism in susceptible subjects (euthyroid patients with Hashimoto's thyroiditis or euthyroid patients previously treated with I-131 or surgery for Graves' disease).

92 CASE STUDIES IN ENDOCRINOLOGY

2. Hypomagnesemia may be associated with hyperthyroidism. A thyrotoxic patient with severe weakness should have serum magnesium, calcium, and potassium measured.

3. The radionuclide thyroidal uptake or scan is not ordered to make a diagnosis of hyperthyroidism but is helpful in deciding the etiology of the hyperthyroidism.

REFERENCES

Blum M, Shenkman L, Hollander CS: The autonomous nodule of the thyroid: correlation of patient age, nodule size, and functional status. Am J Med Sci 269:43, 1975.

DeGroot LJ, Larsen PR, Refetoff S, Stanbury JB: Multinodular goiter. The Thyroid and its Diseases, ed. 5. New York, John Wiley & Sons, 1984, pp 732-755.

Dodd MJ, Blake DR: A case of apathetic thyrotoxicosis simulating malignant disease. Postgrad Med J 56:359, 1980.

Fradkin JE, Wolff J: Iodide-induced thyrotoxicosis. Medicine 62:1, 1983.

Kallee E, Wahl R, Bohner J, et al: Thyrotoxicosis induced by iodine-containing drugs. J Mol Med 4:221, 1980.

Lahey FH: Apathetic thyroidism. Ann Surg 93:1026, 1931.

Peake RL: Recurrent apathetic hyperthyroidism. Arch Int Med 141:258, 1981.

NODULAR THYROID GLAND

CASE 13: B.D., a 28-year-old physical education teacher, presented because of a prominent fullness in his neck. He had noted that his shirt collars were getting tighter over the last year. He thought this discomfort related to increased neck musculature since he lifted weights regularly. Three weeks ago, his friends noted a mass on the right side of his neck. He had experienced no pain, fever, hoarseness, dysphagia, dyspnea, nervousness, weight loss, or diarrhea. There was no prior history of head or neck irradiation nor any family history of endocrine disease.

His weight was 186 lb; height, 72 inches; BP, 125/80; pulse, 80/min. He was a muscular man with the only positive findings limited to the neck. On the right side a 3.5-cm soft mass was located anterior to sternocleidomastoid. The margins were smooth and palpated as part of the right lobe of the thyroid. The mass moved when he swallowed. No other cervical nodules were noted. His eye, skin, and neurological exams were normal.

94 CASE STUDIES IN ENDOCRINOLOGY

ENDOCRINE CLUE: Serum T4(RIA) was 10.9 µg/dl; T3U, 44% (normal, 35-45%). Fine needle aspiration biopsy of the thyroid mass was performed. No fluid was obtained. The cytopathology report read "benign appearing epithelial cells with a few macrophages and scant amount of colloid."

QUESTIONS:

1. What is the most likely diagnosis?

2. The patient was started on thyroid suppression therapy. Exogenous thyroid hormone is administered to suppress the pituitary-thyroid axis, a conventional method to treat thyroid masses not thought to be cancerous. After taking L-thyroxine 0.125 mg/day for 4 weeks, he returned complaining of nervousness, heat intolerance, and palpitations. What studies would you order?

3. Knowing the results of these studies, what is the diagnosis?

4. What would you recommend?

ANSWERS:

1. <u>Colloid nodule (hyperplastic type) versus follicular adenoma</u>. The cytopathology favors the former (follicular adenoma generally have uniform cells with very little colloid being present).

2. The symptoms are compatible with thyrotoxicosis. <u>Order serum T4(RIA) and T3U</u>. *[These values return: T4, 15 µg/dl; T3U, 48%.]* The dose of L-thyroxine prescribed does not normally cause hyperthyroidism. This raises the possibility of autonomous functioning thyroid tissue. Of course, the patient might have thyrotoxicosis factitia (i.e., taking more than prescribed amount of L-thyroxine). <u>Obtaining 24-hour I-131 or I-123 thyroidal uptake and scintiscan provides the answer for both of these possibilities</u>. Here is this patient's thyroid scan:

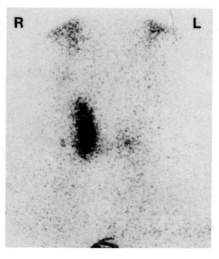

NODULAR THYROID GLAND 97

The 24-hour thyroidal uptake was 26%. Normal uptake varies with the size of the cold iodine pool and ranges between 10 and 30% in the United States. However, <u>while ingesting suppressive amounts of T4 or T3, the 24-hour thyroidal uptake should be less than 5%.</u>

3. <u>Autonomous functioning thyroid nodule.</u> When the nodule produces enough T4 and T3 (often more T3 than T4) to cause hyperthyroidism, the diagnosis would be "toxic adenoma." This patient became toxic due to an additional load of thyroid hormone orally. The scintiscan showed a hyperfunctioning right lobe and decreased activity in the left lobe.

4. First, have the patient stop taking L-thyroxine. Within 2-3 weeks, the hyperthyroid symptoms should abate. If hyperthyroidism persists, then ablative therapy with surgery resection or I-131 is necessary. The author prefers surgical resection of the nodule unless there are extenuating reasons that might prohibit anesthesia and surgery (e.g., an elderly or poor risk patient with cardiac or respiratory compromise). This patient became euthyroid after L-thyroxine was discontinued. Since the risk of future hyperthyroidism was high, this patient had elective thyroid surgery to remove the right lobe of the thyroid.

PEARLS:

1. Toxic adenoma occurs in a younger age group (often in the thirties or forties) than does the toxic multinodular goiter.

2. Many toxic nodules secrete increased amounts of T3 and near-normal amounts of T4, leading to a diagnosis of T3-thyrotoxicosis. <u>It is a good idea to order serum T3(RIA),</u>

98 CASE STUDIES IN ENDOCRINOLOGY

<u>particularly in patients with nodular thyroid glands who might be hyperthyroid.</u>

3. Autonomous thyroid nodules generally do not cause hyperthyroidism until the nodule reaches 3 or more cm in diameter. However, multiple autonomous nodules need not be this size to make the patient thyrotoxic.

4. The surgical pathology of the nodule determines whether postoperative thyroid suppression is recommended. If the nodule is a simple thyroid adenoma without colloid cyst formation, then no treatment is needed. If there is significant colloid formation to suggest a generalized process, then L-thyroxine might be prescribed with the hope of preventing future nodules and thus avoiding surgery.

PITFALLS:

1. <u>Patients with toxic adenoma are not treated with long-term antithyroid medications.</u> These patients need ablative therapy, not suppressive treatment that is doomed to fail as soon as the thionamide is discontinued. Short-term treatment with antithyroid medication is necessary for most patients prior to definitive therapy.

2. If the thyroid scintiscan shows no evidence of function on the side opposite to the "hot" nodule, <u>the possibility of thyroid hemiagenesis exists</u>. Many endocrinologists would recommend TSH administration prior to surgery, followed by a repeat scintiscan to verify the function of the extranodular tissue.

3. Patients who have nodular thyroid glands (i.e., the elderly patient with a multinodular goiter) <u>ought to avoid taking</u>

iodine preparations (kelp, KI expectorants, etc.), since the incidence of iodine-induced hyperthyroidism increases dramatically. Some of these patients become thyrotoxic several weeks after an inorganic iodine load (e.g., amiodarone or radiographic contrast agents). Symptomatic treatment with propranolol and withdrawal of any iodine-containing medication is indicated.

REFERENCES

Bransom CJ, Talbot CH, Henry L, et al: Solitary toxic adenoma of the thyroid gland. Br J Surg 66:590, 1979.

Linfors EW, Neelon FA: Neck masses: illustration of a logical approach. NC Med J 46:574, 1985.

Lividas DP, Koutras DA, Souvatzoglou A, et al: The toxic effects of small iodine supplements in patients with autonomous thyroid nodules. Clin Endocrinol 7:121, 1977.

Mortimer PS, Tomlinson IW, Rosenthal FD: Hemiaplasia of the thyroid with thyrotoxicosis. J Clin Endocrinol Metab 52:152, 1981.

ELDERLY WOMAN WITH DECREASED HEARING

CASE 14: S.N., a 66-year-old widow, complained "I can't hear good." Although she could not date the onset of decreased hearing, she had experienced difficulty listening over the telephone for at least a year. When a daughter who had not seen her mother for 2 years visited her, she noted several things that were unusual for her mother. The house was unkept (her mother had been a compulsive housekeeper) and quite warm (the thermostat was set at 78-80°F during the winter months). Her mother's affect seem to be more jovial and her voice huskier than the daughter had remembered. The patient, however, denied any real changes and had no specific complaints other than decreased hearing. She occasionally had numbness in both hands early in the morning that cleared by 10 AM and at times had some cramping in the calves at night. She denied any constipation (bowel movement every 2-3 days), shortness of breath, use of any medications, or chronic pain. She had been treated with I-131 for hyperthyroidism 15 years ago; no other significant medical or family history was elicited.

This pleasant woman weighed 145 lb; height, 62 inches; BP, 150/100; pulse, regular at 60/min; temperature, 97.8°F. The skin was dry and flaky and had a yellow tinge, particularly over the soles of the feet. HEENT exam showed no cerumen in the auditory canals, normal tympanic membranes, and a Weber test that was nonlateralizing. She did not hear the ticking of a watch held against either pinna. The upper eyelids were puffy (CLUE), and extraocular movements were normal. The tongue was questionably enlarged. Her voice was husky and her speech was slow. The thyroid was not palpable. Neurological exam revealed a woman who moved slowly and who answered questions appropriately, but it took awhile to get the answers. No motor or sensory deficits were found, but there was a delay in the relaxation of the deep tendon reflexes. The remainder of the examination was normal.

ELDERLY WOMAN WITH DECREASED HEARING

ENDOCRINE CLUE: Photograph of the upper part of the patient's face.

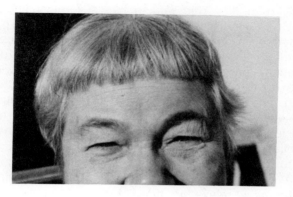

QUESTIONS:

1. What is the most likely diagnosis? Why?

2. What studies should you order to confirm this diagnosis?

3. What are potential causes of this disorder?

4. How would you manage this patient?

5. What are the advantages of prescribing L-thyroxine and the disadvantages of L-triiodothyronine as thyroid replacement?

102　CASE STUDIES IN ENDOCRINOLOGY

ANSWERS:

1. Hypothyroidism. This woman has several findings that are typical of hypothyroidism. Classic symptoms of hypothyroidism include: marked cold intolerance (prefers warm room, extra clothes, sleeps with blanket during the warm months); weakness (increased tiredness, slowing down); muscle cramps, aching, and stiffness; hoarseness, decreased hearing, and paresthesias (a result of myxedematous changes in the vocal cords, middle ear and eighth cranial nerve, and carpal tunnel syndrome); and mental changes (somnolence and dementia). The signs include skin which is rough, scaly, dry, cool to the touch, and pallid or yellow tinted; nonpitting edema of the eyelids; slow movements and slowness of thought; slow relaxation time of deep tendon reflexes; and cardiovascular signs (bradycardia, hypertension). Important tip-offs in this patient include the history of I-131 therapy, the CLUE showing typical finding of upper eyelid edema of hypothyroidism, and the prolonged relaxation phase of the deep tendon reflexes.

2. Hypothyroidism is confirmed by finding a low serum T4(RIA) and T3U. *[This patient's T4 was 2 μg/dl; T3U, 23%.]* Order a serum TSH since the TSH is elevated in all forms of primary hypothyroidism. *[The TSH returned 54 μU/ml (normal, < 6).]*

3. Primary hypothyroidism has several etiologies. Segregating the causes into nongoitrous and goitrous hypothyroidism is helpful clinically. Nongoitrous hypothyroidism includes spontaneous primary thyroid atrophy and postablative hypothyroidism following surgery or radioactive iodine therapy. Goitrous hypothyroidism includes chronic autoimmune thyroiditis (Hashimoto's thyroiditis), drug-induced hypothyroidism (lithium, iodine, or antithyroid drugs), iodine deficiency hypothyroidism (common in endemic areas of the world), and dyshormonogenesis (rare

ELDERLY WOMAN WITH DECREASED HEARING   103

inherited disorders leading to goiter and hypothyroidism). In this patient, postablative hypothyroidism following I-131 caused her disorder.

4. Treatment of primary hypothyroidism is simple: prescribe L-thyroxine in a dose of 2 µg/kg body weight/day (1 µg/lb works well and is easy to remember). The average replacement dose ranges from 100 to 200 µg/day. The regimen for each patient must be individualized. For the elderly and severely hypothyroid patient, gradual initiation of replacement is indicated in order to avoid cardiovascular problems. In this patient, L-thyroxine 0.025 mg/day was prescribed for 2-3 weeks and then increased by 0.025 mg/day every 2-3 weeks until the maintenance dose was reached (L-thyroxine 0.125 mg/day). For the young, mildly hypothyroid patient, one may start with full replacement dose, remembering that it will take nearly a month for the full effects of T4 to be realized. Once the patient is clinically euthyroid, check the serum TSH to make sure it has returned to normal.

5. The half-life of T4 (6 to 8 days) allows for stable and constant serum levels of T4. The advantages of synthetic L-thyroxine include the following: <u>assured potency</u>; <u>single daily dose</u>; <u>inexpensive</u> ($0.06 or less/day); <u>constant levels of serum T4</u>; and the <u>ability to assess adequacy of replacement</u> by measuring serum T4(RIA) for too much replacement or serum TSH for too little supplementation. Most patients normalize their TSH with 0.15 mg of L-thyroxine/day and nearly all with 0.2 mg/day. Since 80% of body T3 is derived by conversion of T4, serum T3(RIA) levels are normal in the patient taking replacement L-thyroxine. T3 is not routinely used for several reasons: peaks of T3 following gut absorption are much higher than normal serum T3(RIA); T3 must be taken three times a day; T3 is considerably more expensive than L-

thyroxine; and serum T4(RIA) cannot be used to assess replacement therapy.

PEARLS:

1. A good schematic to remember regarding control of the thyroid function is given below. TSH secretion is affected by thyrotropin-releasing hormone (TRH) and the nuclear T3 occupancy in the thyrotrope. TRH stimulates TSH release, and high levels of T3 or T4 (via conversion to T3) inhibit TSH release. The thyroidal response to TSH is to increase synthesis and release of T4 (some T3 is also released). Most of the circulating T3 comes from the peripheral conversion of T4 via the ubiquitous 5'-deiodinase that is found in liver, muscle, and other body tissues. T3 (the thyroid metabolite with the most biological activity) and T4 feed back to inhibit TSH secretion.

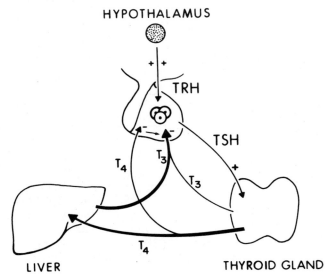

ELDERLY WOMAN WITH DECREASED HEARING   105

2. In hypothyroidism, the tissues are infiltrated by hydrophilic mucopolysaccharides. This leads to the nonpitting edema (most marked in the skin of the eyelids and hands) termed <u>myxedema</u>.

3. <u>Hypothyroidism is often called the "consultant's diagnosis."</u> The subtle and prolonged drift into myxedema may not be appreciated by family, friends, and personal physician.

4. The yellow-tinted skin in Caucasian patients who are hypothyroid relates to hypercarotenemia due to impaired conversion of carotene to vitamin A.

5. Night blindness is not uncommon in hypothyroid patients and is due to decreased synthesis of retinine that is required for dark adaptation.

6. <u>Serum creatine phosphokinase (CPK) is often elevated in untreated hypothyroidism.</u> Decreased clearance of the enzyme probably causes the raised level, since correction of the hypothyroidism causes the level to revert to normal. Serum CPK is not increased in hyperthyroidism.

7. Antibodies to thyroid microsomes and thyroglobulin are usually present in autoimmune thyroid disease (primary atrophy and Hashimoto's thyroiditis). <u>Finding high titers of thyroid antimicrosomal antibodies helps identify the underlying process causing hypothyroidism</u>.

8. Spontaneous hypothyroidism occurs with about one-eighth of the frequency of thyrotoxicosis, but postablative hypothyroidism often follows surgery or radioactive iodine therapy for hyperthyroidism and thus represents the most frequent cause of hypothyroidism.

106 CASE STUDIES IN ENDOCRINOLOGY

9. Muscle aching and cramping (shoulders, upper thighs) are early symptoms of hypothyroidism following surgery or radioactive iodine treatment of hyperthyroidism.

10. Hypothyroid patients may experience deafness and/or vertigo from endolymphatic swelling of the vestibular apparatus (as in this patient).

PITFALLS:

1. Serum T3(RIA) levels do <u>not</u> aid in diagnosing hypothyroidism since over half of the patients with hypothyroidism have serum T3(RIA) values within the normal range.

2. In hypothyroid patients, serum TSH should always be measured; <u>a low TSH level implies pituitary disease.</u>

3. The clinical spectrum of hypothyroidism ranges from subtle and subclinical disease to gross and obvious changes which have developed over years. <u>Do not forget hypothyroidism as a treatable cause of dementia.</u>

4. <u>Primary spontaneous atrophy</u> represents one end of the spectrum of autoimmune thyroid disease; at the other is <u>chronic autoimmune (Hashimoto's) thyroiditis,</u> in which there is marked proliferation of lymphocytes and acinar formation leading to goiter. <u>Remember that there may be failure of other endocrine organs,</u> including pernicious anemia, diabetes mellitus, hypogonadism, hypoparathyroidism, and Addison's disease associated with hypothyroidism.

5. Patients who have a history of thyroid disease and who take iodine-containing expectorants for chronic obstructive

ELDERLY WOMAN WITH DECREASED HEARING 107

pulmonary disease are prime candidates to develop hypothyroidism or hyperthyroidism.

6. Since the metabolism of many drugs is decreased in hypothyroid patients, <u>avoid or use lower dosages for sedatives, tranquilizers, and pain medications.</u> Using medications in normal dosages and not knowing about hypothyroidism may precipitate "myxedema" coma.

REFERENCES

DeGroot LJ, Larsen PR, Refetoff S, Stanbury JB: Adult hypothyroidism. <u>The Thyroid and its Diseases,</u> ed. 5. New York, John Wiley & Sons, 1984, pp 546-609.

Ingbar SH: The thyroid gland. In Wilson JD, Foster DW (eds): <u>Textbook of Endocrinology,</u> ed. 7. Philadelphia, W.B. Saunders Co., 1985, pp 682-815.

Spaulding SW, Utiger RD: The thyroid: physiology, hyperthyroidism, hypothyroidism, and the painful thyroid. In Felig P, Baxter JD, Broadus AE, Frohman LA (eds): <u>Endocrinology and Metabolism.</u> New York, McGraw-Hill, 1981, pp 281-350.

SEVERE HEADACHE AND DECREASED VISION

CASE 15: T.A., a 56-year-old sales clerk, awoke with a severe frontal headache. He had been in good health and rarely had any headaches. Despite four aspirin tablets, his headache intensified. Three hours later he complained of nausea, decreased vision, and a stiff neck. His wife drove him to the emergency room, where he was examined. He appeared lethargic, but responded to questions appropriately. He said that his headache was "the worst he had ever had." There was no history of trauma, hypertension, or exposure to toxins. His review of systems and family history were not helpful.

His BP was 135/70; pulse, 74/min; respiratory rate, 16/min; temperature, 37°C. Visual acuity tested with a Rosenbaum pocket vision screener was 20/200 OD and 20/70 OS. Visual fields by confrontation suggested a temporal field cut OD. The right pupil was 5 mm and responded sluggishly to light; the left pupil was 3 mm and responded briskly to light. Extraocular muscle testing was normal. Blurring of the margins of the optic disk OD was noted. Cranial nerves (excluding cranial nerve II), muscle strength, and deep tendon reflexes were normal. There was questionable nuchal rigidity. The remainder of the exam was normal.

SEVERE HEADACHE AND DECREASED VISION

ENDOCRINE CLUE: Look closely at the sella turcica. Note its size and apparent double floor.

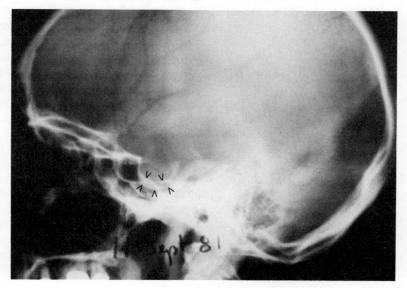

QUESTIONS:

1. What is the most likely diagnosis?

2. What other studies might be performed?

3. What is the treatment for this disorder?

110   CASE STUDIES IN ENDOCRINOLOGY

ANSWERS:

1. Pituitary apoplexy is the most likely diagnosis. Pituitary apoplexy, defined as sudden massive hemorrhage into a pituitary tumor compressing perisellar structures and/or causing signs of meningeal irritation, is an endocrine emergency. Other conditions most commonly considered in the differential diagnosis of sudden headache, ocular signs, and impaired consciousness include aneurysmal subarachnoid hemorrhage and meningitis. Radiological studies help differentiate between apoplexy and aneurysm. The plain X-ray film (see CLUE) demonstrating an enlarged sella turcica strongly supports apoplexy.

2. A CT scan of the pituitary might demonstrate a round, well-defined, high density lesion that has minimal or no enhancement. At times the CT may not exclude an aneursym that mimics a pituitary adenoma causing visual impairment and sella enlargement. An arteriogram is indicated in these cases. Generally, a lumbar puncture does not provide much useful information (erythrocytes might be present in both conditions). Baseline serum studies of endocrine function should be obtained (cortisol, T4 and T3U, testosterone, prolactin).

3. Successful treatment for pituitary apoplexy depends on prompt recognition of the syndrome. Corticosteroid replacement should be started. Doses greater than physiological replacement are used in order to decrease swelling (dexamethasone 10 mg parenterally and 4 mg by mouth every 6 hours). In patients who have lost vision, immediate surgery is almost always required if vision is to be restored. Decompression of the tumor transsphenoidally offers a speedy and less stressful route than does transfrontal craniotomy. After surgery, these patients often

SEVERE HEADACHE AND DECREASED VISION   111

need radiation for residual tumor. Hormone replacement therapy is necessary in nearly all patients.

PEARLS:

1. Generally, pituitary apoplexy is spontaneous. <u>Most patients have no history referable to endocrine deficiency</u>.

2. The manifestations of pituitary apoplexy usually evolves within hours to 2 days. The severity of presentation is generally proportional to the size of the original tumor.

3. Upward enlargement of the adenoma leads to compression of the optic pathways (decreased visual acuity and field defects), diencephalon (dysregulation of temperature, hypotension, and impairment of consciousness), and mesencephalon (motor and respiratory dysfunction).

4. Lateral expansion of the tumor into the cavernous sinus may lead to extraocular ophthalmoplegia (third and then sixth nerves), trigeminal nerve dysfunction (ophthalmic division), venous stasis (proptosis, eyelid swelling), and carotid artery occlusion.

5. Ophthalmoplegia associated with a sellar mass strongly suggests pituitary apoplexy because an uncomplicated pituitary adenoma rarely encroaches into the cavernous sinus.

6. The most reliable CT sign of pituitary apoplexy is the presence of a homogeneous dense lesion showing little or no enhancement or a high density fluid level inside the adenoma.

112   CASE STUDIES IN ENDOCRINOLOGY

7. Not every patient requires surgery, but the clinical course in unpredictable. Those with serious visual or mental impairment require urgent surgical decompression. Ocular palsies are not an absolute surgical indication since they usually resolve spontaneously.

8. Diabetes insipidus (either transient or permanent) is surprisingly rare in pituitary apoplexy.

9. The tumor most frequently identified in pituitary apoplexy is the nonsecretory chromophobe adenoma, followed by prolactinoma.

10. Lateral view of the skull X-ray provides helpful information as to sella size. The sella turcica is enlarged if the length from the most anterior convexity to the most posterior aspect of the sella is > 17 mm and if the height from the floor to a line drawn between the anterior and posterior clinoid processes is > 13 mm.

PITFALLS:

1. Errors in diagnosis of pituitary apoplexy are common. Misdiagnoses include subarachnoid hemorrhage from a ruptured intracranial aneurysm or arteriovenous malformation, stroke, myocardial infarction, migraine, encephalitis, and meningitis.

2. If there is history of sudden headache and evidence of sellar mass <u>without</u> visual defects or ophthalmoplegia, then an arteriogram is needed to rule out an intracranial aneurysm.

3. Not all hemorrhage of the hypophysis relates to hemorrhage/infarction of a pituitary adenoma. Postpartum

SEVERE HEADACHE AND DECREASED VISION 113

hypovolemia, diabetes mellitus, hemolytic crisis, and temporal arteritis are such examples. These conditions are limited to the sella turcica because its unexpanded boundaries prevent compression of parasellar structures. Pituitary hemorrhage or infarction that is limited to the sella may not be clinically symptomatic; evidence for infarction or hemorrhage of pituitary adenomas is a common histological finding.

4. Apoplexy may occur in patients with known pituitary disease (e.g., acromegaly, prolactinoma) following testing of anterior pituitary function with a triple bolus of insulin, gonadotropin-releasing hormone, and thyrotropin-releasing hormone. Pituitary apoplexy is extremely rare following endocrine testing, but it is a condition that needs to be remembered because of its potential fatal outcome.

5. Pituitary apoplexy leaves most patients with hypopituitarism. <u>Every patient needs to carry a medallion or bracelet identifying his or her diagnosis and required medication.</u> Do not forget this practical point.

REFERENCES

Alhajje A, Lambert M, Crabbe J: Pituitary apoplexy in an acromegalic patient during bromocriptine therapy. <u>J Neurosurg</u> 63:288, 1985.

Cardoso ER, Peterson EW: Pituitary apoplexy: a review. <u>Neurosurgery</u> 14:363, 1984.

Chapman AJ, Williams G, Hockley AD, London DR: Pituitary apoplexy after combined test of anterior pituitary function. <u>Br Med J</u> 291:26, 1985.

Laws ER Jr, Ebersold MJ: Pituitary apoplexy—an endocrine emergency. <u>World J Surg</u> 6:686, 1982.

UNDERBITE

CASE 16: F.S., a 43-year-old telephone lineman, came at his dentist's request for the evaluation of underbite and malocclusion. For the last 5 years, his lower jaw had appeared to gradually protrude. His health had been excellent. He denied any symptoms except for an occasional headache and difficulty finding an effective deodorant-antiperspirant. His hat and glove size had not increased. He wore size 11D shoes which had not recently changed. However, he was using a shoe stretcher which he had not previously used. He passed his first and only kidney stone 11 months ago.

His blood pressure was 150/95; pulse, 60/min; height, 69 inches; and weight, 180 lb. His prognathism was mild. Furrowing of the skin was noted over the forehead. The lower incisors were separated more than the upper incisors, leaving gaps between the teeth. The most impressive finding was fullness of the distal phalanges with fleshy finger pads. Several skin tags were present over the posterior chest. Though not visibly enlarged, the thyroid was easily palpable and diffusely enlarged. The remainder of the exam, including visual field testing by confrontation, was normal.

ENDOCRINE CLUE: Fasting plasma glucose was 130 mg/dl; serum calcium, 9.3 mg/dl; serum phosphorus, 4.8 mg/dl.

UNDERBITE 115

QUESTIONS:

1. What is the differential diagnosis?

2. What questions might you ask the patient?

3. What studies would you order?

4. A glucose tolerance test confirms elevated growth hormone levels. What other studies would you perform?

5. Would you recommend any treatment for this patient? If so, what?

116   CASE STUDIES IN ENDOCRINOLOGY

ANSWERS

1. The prognathism suggests three possibilities: **a)** constitutional or familial (e.g., a family history of underbite); **b)** acromegaly; and **c)** acromegaloid syndrome. However, the history (excessive, malodorous perspiration; questionable increase in shoe size; renal stone), physical exam (increased BP, skin furrowing and tags, thyromegaly, acral enlargement), and laboratory studies (increased plasma glucose, hyperphosphatemia) suggest acromegaly or acromegaloid syndrome.

2. Is there a family history of underbite? *[Answer: No.]* Is there a family history of diabetes mellitus? *[No, nor any history of known endocrine disease.]* Even though his glove size was unchanged, how about his ring size? *[His wedding band no longer fits and he cannot wear it.]* Because of thyromegaly, are there any symptoms that suggest hyperthyroidism (other than increased perspiration)? *[No.]* Any family history of renal stones? *[No.]*

3. Acromegaly must be excluded. First, <u>order plasma growth hormone (GH) after an overnight fast</u>. GH levels should be less than 5 ng/ml in men. Because the index of suspicion is so high for acromegaly, an <u>oral glucose tolerance test (GTT) measuring plasma glucose and growth hormone</u> is recommended. <u>Serum somatomedin C</u> (Sm-C) levels are elevated in acromegaly. Many physicians use Sm-C levels as a diagnostic parameter for acromegaly and prefer to follow Sm-C levels as a measure of disease activity in response to treatment. <u>Skull X-ray</u> looking for enlarged frontal sinuses, increased sella turcica size, and prognathism could be helpful (mandatory if GH is elevated). Hand films might show thickening of soft tissues, widening of bones, early osteophyte formation, and tufting and mushrooming of the terminal phalanges.

UNDERBITE 117

4. The results of the GTT were as follows:

Time (hours)	Plasma glucose (mg/dl)	Plasma GH (ng/ml)
0	120	14
1	185	16
2	160	17
3	135	15

The clinical picture and elevated GH levels that do not suppress with glucose make acromegaly the diagnosis. Normal individuals have GH levels that fall below 2 ng/ml during the oral GTT. Evidence for pituitary adenoma should be sought by evaluating for a mass effect (order CT of pituitary and visual fields examination) and assessing loss of other tropic hormones (hypopituitarism). Baseline thyroid function studies and serum testosterone levels are measured. Evaluating the pituitary-adrenal axis with metyrapone testing is generally not done in this situation (see pages 270-271). Occasionally, growth hormone-producing adenomas make prolactin as well (order serum prolactin).

5. The course of acromegaly is insidious and progressive, leading to disfiguration, bony deformity, osteoarthritis, hypertension, diabetes mellitus, and often cardiovascular death. Treatment is indicated to prevent these complications, as well as to ameliorate any mass effect of the pituitary tumor. Treatment consists of neurosurgery or radiation therapy, or often a combination of the two. Although management varies depending on the institution, most pituitary adenomas are treated by transsphenoidal microsurgery. Large pituitary adenomas that extend into the third ventricle are approached by craniotomy. Medical treatment with ergot derivatives (e.g., bromocriptine) and

118   CASE STUDIES IN ENDOCRINOLOGY

somatostatin analogs should be considered as adjunctive therapy.

PEARLS:

1. Examining old photographs of the patient (driver's license, snapshots, etc.) provides helpful information as to diagnosis and rapidity of the clinical course.

2. Growth hormone levels are slightly higher for females than males after an overnight fast (normal males, < 5 ng/ml; normal females, < 10 ng/ml).

3. In patients suspected of having acromegaly, a single blood sample may be obtained 2 hours after a meal. A GH value < 5 ng/ml in females and < 2 ng/ml in males excludes active disease (see Pitfall #4).

4. Acromegalic patients may present complaining only of symptoms of carpal tunnel syndrome. One needs to exclude endocrine causes of carpal tunnel syndrome such as acromegaly and hypothyroidism.

5. Administering thyrotropin-releasing hormone (TRH) does not stimulate GH levels in normal individuals but causes an early rise (15-30 minutes) of GH in 80-90% of the patients with acromegaly. TRH stimulation is particularly helpful in confirming the diagnosis of acromegaly when GH levels are minimally elevated.

6. Patients with acromegaloidism mimic those with acromegaly. Headaches, arthralgias, paresthesias, malodorous skin, and hyperhidrosis are common complaints. Acromegaloid patients often have hypertension, abnormal glucose tolerance, and fibroma molluscum, as well as typically enlarged hands and feet and coarse facial features. However,

UNDERBITE   119

patients with acromegaloidism do not have elevated growth hormone or somatomedin levels.

7. Hyperphosphatemia results because GH increases the renal tubular reabsorption of phosphate. GH stimulates renal 1-α-hydroxylase, which leads to elevated 1,25-dihydroxyvitamin D levels in acromegalic patients. As a result, intestinal absorption of calcium and phosphate is increased. Hypercalciuria occurs in 60% of patients with acromegaly (renal stones are much less frequent). 1,25-Dihydroxyvitamin D levels fall to normal after effective treatment of the acromegaly.

8. Cure rates for acromegaly vary. Some of the variation depends on the criteria for cure. Random GH levels less than 5 ng/ml or GH less than 2 ng/ml on a GTT best define a cure. The higher the growth levels prior to treatment (> 75 ng/ml), the lower the probability of cure regardless of therapy.

9. Reduction of GH ameliorates the glucose intolerance, helps the hypertension, and lessens the coarse features. Soft tissue enlargement decreases, but bony proliferative changes persist (hyperostosis frontalis, prognathism, bony spurring). Visceromegaly, including diffuse goiter, resolves with effective treatment.

PITFALLS:

1. The change in facial features in acromegalic patients is slow and often unnoticed by the patient. Be sensitive when asking and commenting on the coarse features. Use of such terms as elephant skin (marked ridging of the forehead and scalp) and fat lips (large and protruding lips) is best avoided.

120   CASE STUDIES IN ENDOCRINOLOGY

2. When ordering and interpreting GH levels, take note of the time of day and activity of the patient. <u>Any form of stress (exercise, surgery, smoking, etc.) may raise GH</u>. Thus, be cautious in interpreting borderline elevated GH values.

3. An oral GTT in acromegalic patients may show GH levels that paradoxically rise (about one-third of the patients), remain the same, or fall (but not to less than 2 ng/ml).

4. When the clinical picture is typical of acromegaly, do not rule out acromegaly if the basal growth hormone is normal. A few patients with acromegaly may have "normal" growth hormone levels and/or normal sella films. Further studies may demonstrate that GH fails to suppress on oral GTT (normal GH levels suppress to < 2 ng/ml), that GH levels rise in response to TRH, or that Sm-C levels are elevated <u>and</u> there is a pituitary microadenoma on CT scan.

5. Following treatment of acromegaly with conventional pituitary irradiation, it may take 6-18 months for GH levels to reach their nadir. Lowering of GH levels following successful transsphenoidal surgery occurs within days of surgery.

6. Though common in acromegalic patients, prognathism, frontal bossing, and visceromegaly are generally <u>not</u> features of acromegaloidism.

7. Serum T4(RIA) and serum testosterone levels are often low because the concentration of binding proteins is lowered in acromegaly. Thus, <u>low T4s do not necessarily mean hypopituitarism</u>; one needs to assess T3U or free T4 levels before making this diagnosis.

8. Although somatomedin C levels can be helpful in following acromegaly, the bulk of clinical experience relates to GH

determinations, which are generally more available and less expensive than somatomedin C measurements.

9. Rarely, carcinoid tumors and pancreatic islet cell tumors make growth hormone-releasing factor leading to elevated GH levels and enlargement of the sella. These acromegalic patients mimic those who have a growth-hormone secreting pituitary adenoma. Removal of the primary tumor cures the acromegaly. These patients are usually found after pituitary surgery. The diagnosis is suspected because the acromegaly persists or recurs or because of other problems that might arise from the primary tumor.

REFERENCES

Ashcraft MW, Hartzband PI, van Herle, AJ, et al: A unique growth factor in patients with acromegaloidism. J Clin Endocrinol Metab 57:272, 1983.

Daughaday WH: The anterior pituitary. In Wilson JD, Foster DW (eds): Textbook of Endocrinology, ed. 7. Philadelphia, W.B. Saunders Co., 1985, pp 568-613.

Feingold KR, Lorenz TJ: Acromegaly with 'normal' growth hormone levels. West J Med 142:95, 1985.

Melmed S, Braunstein GD, Horvath E, et al: Pathophysiology of acromegaly. Endocr Rev 4:271, 1983.

Mims RB: Pituitary function and growth dynamics in acromegaloidism. J Natl Med Assoc 70:919-923, 1978.

Schuster LD, Bantle JP, Oppenheimer JH, Seljeskog EL: Acromegaly: reassessment of the long-term therapeutic effectiveness of transsphenoidal pituitary surgery. Ann Intern Med 95: 172, 1981.

MILKY BREAST DISCHARGE AND ABSENT MENSES

CASE 17: S.B., a 24-year-old waitress, presented for evaluation of absent menses. Her menstruation began at the age of 11 years and was monthly until the age of 21. At that time, she became pregnant and delivered a healthy full-term infant. She nursed the child for 6 months and resumed menses shortly thereafter. These periods, however, were scant in flow and spaced irregularly from 1 to 3 months apart. For the last 12 months, her menses ceased entirely. She occasionally noticed a milky breast discharge from both nipples, but denied any pain, decreased vision, headache, cold intolerance, or weight change. Family history revealed no endocrine disease.

She weighed 130 lb; height, 66 inches; BP, 110/70; pulse, 76/min. The only positive finding was bilateral galactorrhea elicited with manual expression. HEENT exam, including visual fields to confrontation, was normal. The thyroid was not enlarged. The neurological exam was normal.

ENDOCRINE CLUE: A serum prolactin was drawn and reported to be 90 ng/ml (normal levels, < 20 ng/ml).

QUESTIONS:

1. What conditions cause hyperprolactinemia?

2. Are there any other questions or laboratory studies that might help define this patient's problem?

3. Given the data in response to Question #2, what is this patient's diagnosis?

4. What do you know about the natural history of this disorder?

5. What are the indications for treatment?

6. If she did not wish to be pregnant again, what would you recommend?

7. If she desired pregnancy, what would you recommend?

124   CASE STUDIES IN ENDOCRINOLOGY

ANSWERS:

1. This woman has hyperprolactinemia.   Numerous causes of hyperprolactinemia include:

<u>Neurogenic</u>: thoracic sensory nerve stimulation, suckling or nipple stimulation;
<u>Hypothalamic and interruption of portal circulation</u>: stalk section, granulomatous disease, neoplasms such as craniopharyngioma, pituitary tumors that affect blood flow;
<u>Pituitary</u>: prolactin-secreting adenomas;
<u>Endocrine</u>: pregnancy, estrogen administration, hypothyroidism;
<u>Drugs impairing dopamine secretion and action</u>: psychotropic such as phenothiazines and butyrophenones; antihypertensives (methyldopa, reserpine), antiemetics (metoclopramide, prochlorperazine), H2-blockers (cimetidine), and opiates;
<u>Other causes</u>: chronic renal failure, cirrhosis, carcinomas of lung and kidney.

2. Before any elaborate work-up, some clinical sleuthing is necessary. You ought to ask: <u>Is the patient taking any drugs or medications?</u> *[No.]* <u>Is the patient hypothyroid?</u> *[Not clinically, but order T4(RIA) and T3U; both were normal.]* <u>Is she pregnant?</u> *[Pelvic exam showed no evidence for this, but you order serum beta-HCG. It is negative.]* Because of the likelihood of a prolactin-secreting pituitary adenoma, <u>you order a skull X-ray and a CT scan of the pituitary</u>. The X-ray shows a normal sized sella turcica and configuration (Hardy grade 0).   Hardy's criteria provide a useful radiographic classification of pituitary lesions.

GRADE	SIZE of SELLA	FLOOR
0	Normal	Intact
I	Normal	Focal thinning
II	Enlarged	Intact
III	Enlarged	Focal erosion
IV	Diffuse destruction of sella	

MILKY BREAST DISCHARGE AND ABSENT MENSES   125

[This patient's pituitary CT using enhancement techniques demonstrated no abnormality.]

3. <u>Prolactinoma.</u> Though the CT scan failed to show a problem, this patient probably has a microadenoma (< 1 cm in size). Tumors that are harbored in Hardy grade 0 sellas are rarely demonstrated on CT scan.

4. The radioimmunoassay for prolactin has raised our awareness of this clinical syndrome and has led to an increased frequency of diagnosis. <u>Our understanding of the natural history of prolactinomas continues to evolve.</u> Most patients with untreated hyperprolactinemia have a benign course; that is, most microadenomas show little or no growth or increased secretion over a matter of years. In fact, many of these patients have spontaneous improvement of the hyperprolactinemia. Certainly a few microadenomas progress to macroadenomas, but just how often that occurs is uncertain.

5. There are at least three indications for treatment: **a)** <u>a desire for pregnancy;</u> **b)** <u>macroadenoma</u> (Hardy grades II-IV; neurological signs of mass effect: decreased visual acuity, visual field cuts, cranial nerve palsies, hypopituitarism); and **c)** <u>annoying galactorrhea</u> (e.g., requiring breast pads).

6. Women with microprolactinomas who do not mind amenorrhea or who do not wish to become pregnant can be followed with serum prolactin measurement every 6 to 12 months. Any suggestions of tumor enlargement such as a dramatic increase in serum prolactin or development of neurologic signs would mean further evaluation, including a CT scan of the pituitary. The question of whether these amenorrheic women need estrogen replacement to prevent osteopenia is unanswered. Generally they do not complain of vaginal dryness or other symptoms of hypoestrogenemia.

126   CASE STUDIES IN ENDOCRINOLOGY

Progestin-induced withdrawal bleeding every 3 months is recommended along with adequate oral calcium supplementation (1.0-1.5 gm of elemental calcium/day).

7. There are two options: <u>treatment with bromocriptine</u> or <u>pituitary surgery via transsphenoidal route (TPS)</u>. In this patient there is greater than a 90% chance that an experienced neurosurgeon using TPS can resect the microadenoma, preserve normal pituitary function, and allow reduction of the serum prolactin to normal and resumption of regular menses. Although the morbidity is very low (< 1%), long-term results with TPS show recurrence of tumor in 9-55% of these patients (<u>20% is the average</u>) 5 years after surgery. Since the natural history of most hyper-prolactinemic patients is benign, many physicians use the dopamine agonist bromocriptine 1.25-2.5 mg two to three times a day (starting with 1.25 mg at bedtime to reduce nausea) to lower the prolactin and induce menstruation. Once pregnancy is confirmed, bromocriptine is stopped. Microadenomas rarely enlarge during pregnancy, though careful follow-up is necessary. The author prefers bromocriptine therapy for this patient.

PEARLS:

1. Patients with amenorrhea and serum prolactin levels > 200 ng/ml almost certainly have a prolactin-secreting pituitary adenoma. Often these patients have a macroadenoma.

2. A normal CT scan of the pituitary in a hyperprolactinemic patient suspected of having prolactinoma does not preclude a prolactinoma. Up to 30% of these patients have a prolactinoma found at surgery.

MILKY BREAST DISCHARGE AND ABSENT MENSES 127

3. Small prolactinomas are generally found in the anterior portion of the adenohypophysis. Because the tumor is visible in the operative field, surgical resection (via the transsphenoidal approach) is technically easier than in Cushing's disease, where the tumor is often smaller and embedded within the pituitary (multiple cuts are necessary to identify the tumor).

4. Macroadenomas are generally treated with surgery, though the chance of obtaining normal prolactin levels postoperatively is low (30%). Because the results with surgery are at times disappointing, bromocriptine is often administered. Serum prolactin levels fall while bromocriptine is taken, and occasionally there is a dramatic reduction of tumor size. Unfortunately, most patients relapse as soon as the bromocriptine is discontinued. Often, bromocriptine is used prior to surgical intervention.

5. Men with prolactinomas present with impotence and hypogonadism. These patients generally have large tumors causing mass effects and hypopituitarism.

PITFALLS:

1. A major drawback of chronic bromocriptine administration is cost ($0.55-0.80/2.5-mg tablet); another is the invariable relapse that follows after bromocriptine is withdrawn.

2. The **References** include articles that show excellent results with TPS or with long-term bromocriptine treatment, but future studies of efficacy of therapy should include an untreated control group that is randomly selected and concomitantly followed.

128 CASE STUDIES IN ENDOCRINOLOGY

REFERENCES

Charpentier G, dePlunkett T, Jedynak P, et al: Surgical treatment of prolactinoma: short- and long-term results and prognostic factors. Hormone Res 22:222, 1985.

Clayton RN, Webb J, Heath PA, et al: Dramatic and rapid shrinkage of a massive invasive prolactinoma with bromocriptine: a case report. Clin Endocrinol 22: 573, 1985.

Corenblum B, Taylor PJ: Long-term follow-up of hyperprolactinemic women treated with bromocriptine. Fertil Steril 40:596, 1983.

Daughaday WH: The anterior pituitary. In Wilson JD, Foster DW (eds): Textbook of Endocrinology, ed. 7. Philadelphia, W.B. Saunders Co., 1985, pp 568-613.

Koppelman MCS, Jaffe MJ, Rieth KG, et al: Hyperprolactinemia, amenorrhea, and galactorrhea: a retrospective assessment of twenty-five cases. Ann Intern Med 100:115; 1984.

March CM, Kletzkey OA, Davajan V, et al: Longitudinal evaluation of patients with untreated prolactin-secreting pituitary adenomas. Am J Obstet Gynecol 139:835, 1981.

Melmed S, Braunstein GD, Chang RJ, Becker DP: Pituitary tumors secreting growth hormone and prolactin. Ann Intern Med 105:238, 1986.

Randal RV, Laws ER Jr, Abboud CF, et al: Transsphenoidal microsurgical treatment of prolactin-producing pituitary adenomas: results in 100 patients. Mayo Clin Proc 58:108,1983.

Thomson JA, Teasdale GM, Gordon D, et al: Treatment of presumed prolactinoma by transsphenoidal operation: early and late results. Br Med J 291:1550, 1985.

EXCESSIVE THIRST AND POLYURIA

CASE 18: D.G., a 57-year-old secretary, was referred from the psychiatry clinic for evaluation of excessive thirst and polyuria. For at least 10 years she had complained of dry mouth and increased thirst that was temporarily relieved by ice water. She drank at least 7 liters of liquid each day. When taking long trips in her automobile, she carried a cooler containing a least of liter of beverage. Every night she got up to urinate at least five times and drank a glass of water on each occasion. Her general health had been good with no history of weight loss, cough, head trauma, or stroke. She had been diagnosed as having a manic-depressive disorder 5 years ago and had been treated with lithium chloride and perphenazine. She did not drink beer or alcohol. The family history was negative for any endocrine disorder.

She weighed 117 lb; height, 59 inches; BP, 140/80; pulse, 60/min and regular. The physical examination was completely normal.

130 CASE STUDIES IN ENDOCRINOLOGY

ENDOCRINE CLUE: Serum electrolytes: Na, 140 mEq/l; K, 3.7 mEq/l; BUN, 13 mg/dl; glucose, 86 mg/dl; Ca, 9.7 mg/dl. Urinalysis: specific gravity, 1.002; no glucose, protein, or cells found.

QUESTIONS:

1. What are the possible causes of this patient's polydipsia and polyuria? Which is most likely?

2. What is the role of lithium in this patient's symptoms?

3. What studies would you order to work up this problem?

4. How would you perform a water deprivation test?

5. After reviewing the data (Question #4), what is the diagnosis?

6. Is any further workup indicated?

7. What would you recommend for therapy?

132   CASE STUDIES IN ENDOCRINOLOGY

ANSWERS:

1. The possible causes include <u>neurogenic diabetes insipidus</u>, <u>nephrogenic diabetes insipidus</u>, or <u>primary polydipsia</u> (psychogenic or compulsive water drinker). Diabetes mellitus was easily excluded by the absence of glycosuria and elevated blood sugar. Because this patient had a long history of polydipsia and polyuria and had known affective disorder, primary polydipsia seems most likely. A note of caution, however: these polydipsic patients often are mildly hyponatremic, reflecting chronic volume overload, a condition which this patient did not have.

2. Therapeutic levels of lithium cause nephrogenic diabetes insipidus in up to one-third of patients. The kidneys' ability to concentrate urine usually returns within a month after the lithium is stopped. Although lithium might contribute to this patient's symptoms, the polyuria and polydipsia antedated the lithium therapy by several years, making lithium an unlikely primary culprit.

3. A method to assess renal handling of water is necessary. The ideal study would measure plasma and urine osmolality and correlate these values with serum vasopressin or antidiuretic hormone (ADH) levels. Inappropriately dilute urine in a patient with hypertonic serum and nonmeasureable ADH levels would be diagnostic of neurogenic diabetes insipidus. Under the same circumstances, a high level of ADH indicates nephrogenic diabetes insipidus. Since vasopressin levels are available in only a few centers, dehydration is used as the biological assay to assess the action of ADH on the kidney. ADH concentrates urine by making the collecting tube permeable to water. In the absence of ADH, urine is dilute and its osmolality low. <u>Order a water deprivation-ADH study for this patient</u>.

EXCESSIVE THIRST AND POLYURIA 133

4. The dehydration test must be carefully performed and the patient closely monitored. If the history suggests significant polyuria (as in this patient), then total fluid restriction is begun at 8-9 AM after baseline body weight and urine and plasma osmolality are determined. In cases of less severe polyuria, total fluid restriction may begin earlier (at bedtime) after the same baseline variables are measured. <u>Use a flow sheet to record responses</u>. The flow sheet should have the following headings: time, body weight, urine specific gravity (a convenient bedside monitor of urine osmolality), urine volume, and urine and plasma osmolality. Body weight and urine values are assessed hourly. When the urine osmolality stabilizes (specific gravity unchanged at the bedside and the laboratory confirms that the hourly increase in urine osmolality is < 30 mOsm/kg for 3 hours), then blood is drawn for plasma osmolality. A plasma value > 288 mOsm/kg assures adequate dehydration. The following table shows the results of this patient's water deprivation-ADH study.

TIME (hr)	WEIGHT (lb)	URINE			SERUM OSMOLALITY (mOsm/kg)
		Volume (ml)	Sp Gr	Osmolality (mOsm/kg)	
0900	119		1.004	131	282
1000	119	350	1.003	125	283
1100	118	400	1.003	172	285
1200	117	300	1.002	150	287
Aqueous vasopressin 5 U given sc at 1200					
0100	117	90	1.007	280	287
0200	117	40	1.016	520	287

Some patients will surreptitiously imbibe water during the study and thus will not concentrate their urine. After urine osmolality stabilizes, aqueous vasopressin 5 U is given subcutaneously, and urine and plasma osmolality are

134 CASE STUDIES IN ENDOCRINOLOGY

measured 1 hour later. If body weight decreases below 3% of the initial weight, then the test is stopped _after_ the plasma and urine osmolalities are measured and the response to aqueous vasopressin is performed.

5. This patient failed to increase her urine osmolality when deprived of water. The normal response results in a urine osmolality two to four times that of plasma. After administration of aqueous pitressin, her urine volume decreased dramatically, and the urine osmolality increase significantly. Patients with neurogenic diabetes insipidus have urine osmolalities that rise > 150 mOsm/kg in response to aqueous vasopressin. Normal subjects and those with nephrogenic diabetes insipidus have little or no rise in urine osmolality (< 9% increase) in response to vasopressin. Some difficulty in interpreting this test arises in those patients with diabetes insipidus who have residual capacity to secrete ADH under the hypertonic conditions of the dehydration test and in compulsive water drinkers who have diluted the concentration gradient in the renal medulla such that even high levels of ADH cannot produce a normally concentrated urine during the short interval of this test. In these circumstances the clinical assessment is important. If there is still doubt regarding the diagnosis, then the plasma from the dehydration test should be assayed for vasopressin. In diabetes insipidus (neurogenic) the plasma vasopressin will be low, whereas vasopressin levels will be appropriately elevated in primary polydipsia. _This patient meets the criteria for complete neurogenic diabetes insipidus._

6. Yes. Careful evaluation for neoplasms of the pituitary and hypothalamus is mandatory. Neurogenic diabetes insipidus has several possible etiologies: idiopathic (about 30% of cases), tumors of brain or pituitary fossa (25%), head trauma (15%), following cranial surgery for tumor or hypophysectomy (20%), and other causes (granulomatous

EXCESSIVE THIRST AND POLYURIA 135

diseases including sarcoidosis and eosinophilic granuloma). Order a CT scan of the pituitary. *[CT was normal.]* The long history of polydipsia and polyuria and the negative CT scan suggest "idiopathic" disease.

7. After the diagnosis of diabetes insipidus is firmly established, there are several methods of controlling the polyuria. If the thirst mechanism is intact, as it usually is, then taking vasopressin is a matter of convenience to avoid having to drink excessively and urinate frequently. Specific treatment is available using vasopressin. The most inexpensive form of ADH is vasopressin tannate (5 U/ml). A 1-ml injection of this oil suspension given intramuscularly lasts for 2 to 4 days and costs $1.00 to $1.50. Complications include sterile abscesses and hypertension. Patients with hypertension and those who do not like injections may take desmopressin (DDAVP) 0.05-0.15 ml once or twice per day. This medication is absorbed through the nasal mucosa by blowing the solution out of a cannula directed into the nares. Cost is a factor (up to $2000/year). Lysine vasopressin nasal spray is effective but must be used at frequent intervals (every 3 to 6 hours).

Nonhormonal oral agents are effective in controlling the polyuria. The advantages of these agents is that they are easy to administer, cost less, and provide smoother and more predictable control. Chlorpropamide 250-500 mg each day invariably reduces urine volume about 50%, but there is considerable variation among patients. When urine volume cannot be reduced to asymptomatic levels, addition of a thiazide diuretic often helps. Of course, hypoglycemia is the dreaded side effect. Calorie restriction and severe exercise should be avoided with this treatment. Patient with anterior pituitary compromise and those who are pregnant should not be given chlorpropamide. Thiazide diuretics have a paradoxical effect of reducing urine output in patients with

136 CASE STUDIES IN ENDOCRINOLOGY

diabetes insipidus. If chlorpropamide 500 mg each day and hydrochlorothiazide 25 mg twice a day do not achieve satisfactory control or if unmanageable side effects occur, then the patient is treated with desmopressin.

PEARLS:

1. Normal (ad lib water) plasma osmolality ranges between 270 and 290 mOsm/kg. If the plasma osmolality and serum sodium are > 295 mOsm/kg and > 143 mEq/l, respectively, under conditions of ad lib fluid intake, the diagnosis of primary polydipsia is excluded.

2. A significant increase in urine output immediately after pituitary surgery usually indicates diabetes insipidus, but diabetes mellitus must be excluded. Replacement with intravenous fluid in amounts equivalent to urine output is justified for several hours. Then, reduce the intravenous rate for for 1-2 hours and check the serum and urine osmolality. A plasma osmolality above 287 mOsm/kg insures volume contraction and excludes volume overload as the cause of the diuresis. Aqueous vasopressin 5 U is given subcutaneously. If the patient has diabetes insipidus, both the urine volume and serum osmolality should decrease over next hour in response to vasopressin.

3. Urine volume > 18 liters/day, plasma osmolality < 280 mOsm/kg, absence of nocturia, or episodic polyuria suggest compulsive water drinking as the underlying disorder.

4. Chlorpropamide, carbamazepine, and clofibrate may be used to treat neurogenic diabetes insipidus, but are totally ineffective in reducing the urine volume of nephrogenic diabetes insipidus.

EXCESSIVE THIRST AND POLYURIA   137

5. In contrast to diabetes insipidus that develops immediately following minor head trauma, most patients with delayed onset of diabetes insipidus after trauma have permanent ADH deficiency.

6. Familial nephrogenic diabetes insipidus occurs as a rare X-linked syndrome with resistance to ADH. <u>Drug-induced nephrogenic diabetes insipidus</u> is much more common; <u>demeclocycline, methyoxyflurane, and lithium are the classic offenders</u>.

PITFALLS:

1. Treatment of anterior pituitary deficiency of ACTH and/or TSH with glucocorticoids and/or thyroxine may unmask partial diabetes insipidus and precipitate polyuria. Similarly, if polyuria does not recur following discontinuation of ADH supplementation in neurosurgical patients treated for diabetes insipidus, then consider concomitant deficiency of ACTH or TSH as well as transient diabetes insipidus.

2. One should be aware of the triphasic response of diuresis-antidiuresis-diuresis after pituitary or hypothalamic injury. One to two days postoperatively, there is a diuresis that lasts for 3-5 days (probably due to neurohypophyseal trauma), then amelioration for 4-5 days (due to release of stored ADH granules), followed by full-blown diuresis (the sequela of permanent injury).

3. <u>Hypertonic saline infusions are hazardous</u> and are best avoided. The water deprivation-ADH test defines patients with severe neurogenic diabetes insipidus or nephrogenic

138 CASE STUDIES IN ENDOCRINOLOGY

diabetes insipidus. Plasma ADH levels are most helpful in distinguishing partial or incomplete diabetes insipidus.

4. Never prescribe vasopressin tannate (an oil preparation) for the acute stage of polyuria. Use aqueous vasopressin or DDAVP initially until the diagnosis of diabetes insipidus is confirmed. Never prescribe ADH for primary polydipsia; dilutional hyponatremia and seizures are likely to follow.

REFERENCES

Case records of Massachusetts General Hospital, Case 5-1985. N Engl J Med 312:297, 1985.

Culpepper RM, Hebert SC, Androli TE: The posterior pituitary and water metabolism. In Wilson JD, Foster DW (eds): Textbook of Endocrinology, ed. 7. Philadelphia, W.B. Saunders, 1985, pp 614-652.

Handani M, Findler G, Skaked I, et al: Unusual delayed onset of diabetes insipidus following closed head trauma. J Neurosurg 63:456, 1985.

Kern KB, Meislin HW: Diabetes insipidus: occurrence after minor head trauma. J Trauma 24:69, 1984.

Milles JJ, Spruce B, Baylis PH: A comparison of diagnostic methods to differentiate diabetes insipidus from primary polyuria: a review of 21 patients. Acta Endocrinol 104:410, 1983.

Weiss NM, Robertson GL: Diabetes insipidus. In Krieger DT, Bardin CW (eds): Current Therapy in Endocrinology 1985-1986. Toronto, B.C. Decker, 1985, pp 1-3.

IMPOTENCE

CASE 19: B.C., a 56-year-old business executive, complained that he could not have sex. For the last year his penile erections failed to reach full tumescence so that he could not engage in intercourse. Over the past month, he has had no erections, including the lack of early morning erections. He denied any prior history of sexual difficulty, any problems with his wife, job, or family, or history of any medical problems. He took no medications and did not drink alcohol or smoke tobacco. His review of systems was negative for persistent headache, loss of visual acuity, and claudication or paresthesias in the lower extremities. He had, however, noted that his beard growth had diminished. He shaved every other day where previously he would shave daily.

He weighed 177 lb; height, 72 inches; BP, 130/85; pulse, 78/min and regular. He appeared healthy. HEENT, chest, and abdominal exams were normal. His testes were of normal size (3.0 x 5.0 cm bilaterally) and consistency. The prostate was slightly enlarged but not tender. His extremities had good distal arterial pulsations. The neurological exam was normal.

140 CASE STUDIES IN ENDOCRINOLOGY

ENDOCRINE CLUE: The combination of absence of penile erections and a change in shaving frequency suggests a significant underlying cause.

QUESTIONS:

1. What factors affect potency?

2. What factors affect the penile erectile mechanism?

3. What screening studies would you order in this patient?

4. After reviewing the data (Answer #3), what is this patient's diagnosis?

5. How should this patient be managed?

6. How would you treat his chronic hypogonadism?

142   CASE STUDIES IN ENDOCRINOLOGY

ANSWERS:

1. Potency, the ability to achieve or to maintain a penile erection which will allow the patient to engage in coitus, is affected by <u>libido and physical health</u>. <u>Libido</u>, the physiologic and mental drive for sexual satisfaction, varies among individuals and within each individual. Libido is influenced by social and sexual experiences, physical and mental illness, and medication. Drugs that diminish libido include alcohol, tranquilizers, antidepressants, sedatives, opiates, antihypertensives, and estrogens. Hypogonadism also affects libido. Furthermore, <u>potency depends on normal anatomy and physiologic function.</u>

2. The erectile mechanism requires intact <u>neurologic</u>, <u>vascular</u>, and <u>endocrine</u> systems. Impairment of any one of these can produce impotence.

Neurogenic impotence: Any disruption of the parasympathetic autonomous nervous system impairs erectile ability. Stimulation of the S2-S4 nerve roots via the nervi erigentes causes relaxation of specialized vascular smooth muscles ("polsters") leading to engorgement of the corpora cavernosa. Many diseases interfere with parasympathetic outflow: diabetes mellitus, alcoholism, heavy metal intoxication, cord tumors, and multiple sclerosis. Surgical procedures such as prostatectomy or retroperineal dissection may impair the erectile mechanism.

Vascular impotence: Full erection requires adequate penile blood flow. Obstruction of the aorta, iliac vessels, or hypogastric or pudendal arteries can lead to impotence. <u>Leriche's syndrome</u> provides a good example (lower extremity claudication and impotence). Small arteriole disease associated with diabetes mellitus also causes impotence.

IMPOTENCE 143

Anatomic impotence: Genitourinary conditions such as Peyronie's disease, urethritis, severe chordee, and penile trauma may result in impotence.

Endocrine impotence: The hormonal milieu must be adequate for potency. Normal adrenal and thyroid functions are important to male sexual function, but the testosterone production is paramount. Testosterone stimulates protein synthesis (muscle mass) and virilization (enlargement of the phallus, scrotal rugosity and pigmentation, and hair growth on the face, chest, and back). High intratesticular levels of testosterone are essential to normal spermatogenesis. Testosterone also affects the limbic system (and thus libido). Testosterone deficiency (hypogonadism) is an important cause of endocrine impotence and is most amenable to treatment.

3. Determination of serum testosterone, serum luteinizing hormone (LH), and serum prolactin usually detects most endocrine causes of impotence. Serum testosterone should be measured in each impotent patient. *[This patient's serum testosterone was 230 ng/dl (normal, 300-1000 ng/dl).]* Since testosterone production is controlled by LH, any disturbance of the hypothalamic-pituitary-testicular axis may lead to testosterone deficiency and impotence. In primary testicular disease, the serum LH is very helpful since it is elevated in the absence of the negative feedback of testosterone. *[Patient's serum LH was 2 mIU/ml (normal, 4-15 mIU/ml).]* Secondary hypogonadism is often due to a prolactinoma which usually presents late (macroadenoma) with impotence being the predominant clinical symptom. Serum prolactin should be ordered if anything suggests hypogonadism in the middle- and late-aged male. *[This patient's serum prolactin was 1250 ng/ml (normal, < 20 ng/ml).]*

144　CASE STUDIES IN ENDOCRINOLOGY

4. <u>Secondary hypogonadism due to a prolactin-secreting pituitary adenoma</u>. Skull series showed an enlarged sella turcica. CT of the pituitary showed a poorly enhancing lesion that filled the entire sella without suprasellar extension. Goldmann perimetry exam showed normal visual fields. Baseline endocrine studies except for pituitary-testicular axis were normal (serum AM cortisol, T4, T3U).

5. <u>Treatment of a macroprolactinoma is not totally successful</u>. Transsphenoidal pituitary resection (TPS) and/or long-term administration of bromocriptine is indicated (see page 126) This patient had TPS. Postoperatively, his serum prolactin was 200 ng/dl. Further treatment with Cobalt-60 irradiation to the sella area was recommended.

6. His hypogonadism was managed with <u>testosterone therapy</u>. Testosterone replacement is simple, effective, and safe. Esterified derivatives of testosterone are given intramuscularly, which assures constant levels necessary to maintain muscle mass, beard growth, and libido. <u>Testosterone cypionate or testosterone enanthate 200 mg intramuscularly every 2-4 weeks restores potency in most hypogonadal males</u>. Replacement is continued indefinitely.

PEARLS:

1. Recurrent or persistent impotence (as opposed to occasional episodes of "honeymoon" impotence) is a considerable problem. Impotence increases with age, so that approximately 20% of the males at age 60 years and 50% of the males at age 70 years are impotent.

2. Libido tends to decrease with age, but <u>loss of sexual interest and drive is most commonly situational</u>. Men may experience

IMPOTENCE 145

dissatisfaction with their accomplishments, frustration, fatigue from overwork, or discouragement and a lack of communication with their sexual partner. These factors, as well as depression and neurosis, account for most impotence in younger men, so-called psychogenic or functional impotence. Appropriate evaluation and counseling as to the pathophysiology of impotence and to the factors that affect libido are necessary in treating these patients.

3. The history is important in evaluating impotence. Drugs, particularly antihypertensive medications, often cause impotence. The patient who can sometimes have normal erections and yet be impotent at other times most likely has functional or psychogenic impotence. Normal erections imply that the neurogenic, vascular, and endocrine systems are intact.

4. The physical examination may give clues about hypogonadism. Anosmia suggests hypogonadotropic hypogonadism (Kallman's syndrome). Visual field cuts point to pituitary disease. Melanosis suggests Addison's disease or hemachromatosis. Small, pea-sized testes that are firm are typical of Klinefelter's syndrome.

5. Klinefelter's syndrome (primary testicular failure due to chromatin-positive gonadal dysgenesis) is a common cause of hypogonadism that affects 1 out of 500 males. Many of these patients develop secondary sex characteristics during puberty since the Leydig cells have not yet involuted.

6. The skin of the chronic hypogonadal male is smooth and soft with crows-foot wrinkles about the eyes and mouth.

7. Patients with primary hypogonadism have low serum testosterone levels and high serum LH levels.

146   CASE STUDIES IN ENDOCRINOLOGY

8. The most common cause of organic impotence (excluding medications) is <u>diabetes mellitus</u>. This is usually due to a combination of vascular obstruction as the result of arteriosclerosis and autonomic neuropathy. An occasional diabetic may have primary testicular failure which produces impotence. Because hypogonadism is treatable, one should measure the level of serum testosterone.

9. The hypogonadotropic impotent patient with diabetes mellitus may well have hemachromatosis. That suspicion would be heightened if liver function studies were abnormal. In this situation, order serum ferritin and transferrin saturation. Hemachromatosis (prevalence, 3 per 1000) remains a neglected diagnosis.

10. If the patient is not hypogonadal yet still has organic impotence (e.g., diabetes mellitus), mechanical devices such as an inflatable prosthesis provide effective therapy for impotence.

11. Occasionally patients with hyperthyroidism present with impotence. The serum testosterone is elevated (> 1200 ng/ml) because hyperthyroidism increases the sex hormone binding globulin (the free testosterone concentration is normal). Treatment of the hyperthyroidism usually corrects the impotence.

12. Testosterone production decreases with age and serum testosterone levels are slightly decreased, but remain well within the normal range.

13. The prevalence of impotence vastly exceeds that of all endocrine disorders. Therefore, <u>most instances of sexual dysfunction are not related to a primary endocrine problem</u>. Probably the most accurate means of distinguishing psychogenic from other causes of impotence is to monitor

IMPOTENCE   147

nocturnal penile tumescence (diminished or absent in most organic impotence).

PITFALLS:

1. There is some diurnal variation in the serum testosterone; the highest levels occur between 6 and 9 AM with a 15-40% decrement by late afternoon. The lower values are still well within the normal range, so a single determination is usually sufficient for diagnostic purposes. More accurate assessment of testosterone levels requires pooling of blood obtained over several intervals (e.g., three samples drawn 20 minutes apart).

2. Normal-sized testes (4.5 $\pm$ 1.0 cm long and 2.5 $\pm$ 0.5 cm wide) do not exclude hypogonadism. <u>Most testicular volume relates to spermatogenesis (seminiferous tubules) and not to testosterone production (Leydig cells)</u>.

3. Failure to virilize by the mid to late teens implies pituitary or gonadal abnormality which must be thoroughly investigated.

4. Testosterone replacement may not restore potency if serum prolactin levels remain significantly elevated after treatment of prolactinoma.

5. Orally administrated alkylated testosterone derivatives are <u>not</u> used to treat chronic hypogonadism because their effects on potency are not predictable and there are risks of hepatotoxicity with long-term therapy.

6. Androgen treatment of patients with functional impotence is <u>not</u> helpful. Several studies have shown that the effect of

148   CASE STUDIES IN ENDOCRINOLOGY

testosterone in these patients matches that of placebo therapy alone. Chronic testosterone treatment of eugonadal males decreases sperm count and testicular volume, so this is not even a good placebo drug.

REFERENCES

Burch WM: Impotence. Consultant 22:275, 1982.

Fairbanks VF, Baldus WP: Hemochromatosis: the neglected diagnosis. Mayo Clin Proc 61:296, 1986.

Karacan I: Diagnosis of erectile impotence in diabetes mellitus. An objective and specific method. Ann Intern Med 92:334, 1980.

Schwartz MF, Kolodny RC, Masters WH: Plasma testosterone levels of sexually functional and dysfunctional men. Arch Sex Behav 9:355, 1980.

Smith KD: Testicular function in the aging male. In DeGroot LJ (ed): Endocrinology. New York, Grune & Stratton, 1979, pp 1577-1581.

Spark RF, White RA, Connolly PB: Impotence is not always psychogenic. Newer insights into hypothalamic-pituitary-gonadal dysfunction. JAMA 243:750, 1980.

Williams TC, Frohman LA: Hypothalamic dysfunction associated with hemochromatosis. Ann Intern Med 103:550, 1985.

HIRSUTISM

CASE 20:   F.K., a 20-year-old beautician, presented for evaluation of increased hair over her upper lip, chin, and sideburn area.   Other areas (around the breast areola, between the breasts, and over the thighs) also troubled her.   The hair growth had become more noticeable over the last 7 years.   For cosmetic reasons, she "plucked" the facial hairs and occasionally shaved her face.   Her menses began at age 12, occurred monthly for a year, then became progressively irregular in frequency, and ceased entirely for the last year.   She had no prior health problems and was taking no medications.   Family history revealed that a paternal aunt had "a large amount of facial hair."

On examination, this fair-complected female weighed 145 lb; height, 63 inches; and BP, 115/65.   Terminal hair over the face, mid-anterior chest, linea alba (extending up from the mons pubis), and thighs was easily recognized.   The skin was otherwise normal (no striae, no temporal balding or hairline recession, only a few acne scars).   No breast discharge could be expressed. The external genitalia were normal.   On bimanual pelvic exam, adnexal masses were palpable.

150   CASE STUDIES IN ENDOCRINOLOGY

ENDOCRINE CLUE: *(Left panel)* Sonogram taken at level of both ovaries. *(Right panel)* Close up view of right ovary.

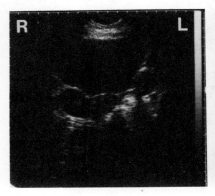 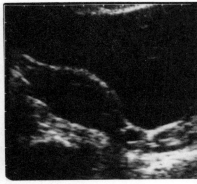

QUESTIONS:

1. What is the most likely diagnosis?

2. Which laboratory studies are appropriate to order to support this diagnosis?

3. What is the current theory regarding the self-perpetuating nature of this disorder?

4. What metabolic events occur at the androgen-sensitive hair follicle that leads to hair growth?

5. What is the treatment for this patient?

6. What general recommendations about therapy would you give to this patient?

152   CASE STUDIES IN ENDOCRINOLOGY

ANSWERS:

1. <u>Polycystic ovary disease is the most likely diagnosis.</u> Most women who present with hirsutism do not have any ominous cause but rather fit into a spectrum of syndromes associated with normal or modestly elevated serum testosterone and elevated free testosterone. These patients have varying degrees of ovarian stromal hyperplasia. Polycystic ovary disease (PCOD) is by far the most common variant. PCOD has its onset just after menarche. It is characterized by chronic anovulation (amenorrhea/oligomenorrhea and dysfunctional uterine bleeding) and slowly progressive hirsutism. A familial tendency may be noted for similar problems. Many patients are obese. Some women have no hirsutism but present for evaluation of infertility. Enlarged ovaries are palpable in about half of the subjects. The pelvic sonogram shows bilateral cystic ovaries in this patient (CLUE).

2. The following laboratory studies are needed to evaluate this patient's hirsutism: <u>serum testosterone, free testosterone (if available), urine 17-ketosteroids or serum dehydro-3-epiandrosterone sulfate (DHEA-S), and serum luteinizing hormone (LH) and follicle stimulating hormone (FSH).</u> If Cushing's syndrome cannot be excluded clinically, collect a 24-hour urine for free cortisol or perform an overnight dexamethasone study (see page 4). Serum testosterone is usually elevated (> 80 ng/dl but < 200 ng/dl), but if not, the serum free testosterone is. Urine 17-ketosteroids and serum DHEA-S are normal or minimally elevated. The ratio of LH to FSH is often elevated (LH/FSH > 2.5). In regard to amenorrhea, pregnancy should be excluded with a <u>serum HCG</u>. When galactorrhea or amenorrhea is present, a serum prolactin is indicated.

3. <u>There is a self-perpetuating cycle of hormonal events associated with polycystic ovaries</u>. Increased ovarian

HIRSUTISM   153

production of testosterone blocks follicular maturation, leading to numerous follicles in varying stages of development. These follicles have limited growth potential and undergo atresia, leading to an increase in the stromal compartment. The stroma normally secretes significant amounts of <u>testosterone</u> and <u>androstenedione</u> and its increased mass results in secretion of a greater amount of androgen. Peripheral conversion of androstenedione into <u>estrone</u> sensitizes the pituitary gonadotrope (as normally happens with increased estrogen levels prior to midcycle LH surge) to respond to gonadotropin-releasing hormone (GnRH), leading to <u>LH production</u>. Estrone also negatively feeds back on FSH production, causing an increased LH/FSH ratio. LH stimulates the ovarian stroma to produce more testosterone (which stimulates hair growth and blocks ovarian follicular maturation, leading to atresia, etc.) and androstenedione (which is converted to estrone and leads to more LH production, etc.). What triggers the cycle is unknown, but recent evidence points to a hypothalamic defect in GnRH-LH regulation.

4. <u>Hair growth in androgen-sensitive areas of the body results from the metabolism of androgens locally at the hair follicle</u>. Increased circulating levels of free testosterone lead to binding of testosterone with androgen receptors at follicles of thin vellus hair. The testosterone-receptor interaction stimulates 5-α-reductase, which converts testosterone to dihydrotestosterone (DHT), a very potent androgen responsible for proliferation and growth of thick terminal hair. Once 5-α-reductase is induced by testosterone, other less potent androgens (such as DHEA and androstenedione) may serve as substrates for the enzyme leading to DHT formation. This system allows for a <u>multiplier effect,</u> in that weaker androgens now become potent steroids because they lead to local production of DHT within the hair follicle. The metabolism of testosterone at the hair follicle may be

154 CASE STUDIES IN ENDOCRINOLOGY

associated with a fall of serum testosterone levels despite continued hair growth.

5. <u>Treatment of PCOD is directed at suppression of ovarian production of androgens using oral contraceptive agents</u>. Ortho-Novum® 2 mg and Demulen® have had wide use for treating PCOD. Ortho-Novum 2 mg is started on the fifth day of menses, and is given for 21 days and repeated cyclically. After 2 to 3 months of treatment, androgens levels are remeasured. If these results are normal or if there has been > 50% reduction, treatment is continued, realizing that any amelioration of the hirsutism will be gradual with a maximal therapeutic effect after 9-12 months. The usual precautions related to oral contraceptives (blood pressure, venous thrombosis, etc.) are necessary. Weight reduction should be encouraged if the patient is overweight. Clomiphene may be used to induce ovulation in those patients who desire pregnancy. Ovarian wedge resection reduces the stromal compartment and may benefit patients who fail to ovulate with clomiphene. Pulsatile GnRH has also been used in patients who desire pregnancy and who fail with clomiphene.

6. <u>Medical therapy is notoriously unsatisfactory in treating hirsutism</u>. Suppression of hyperandrogenism with oral contraceptives, administration of glucocorticoids for congenital adrenal hyperplasia, and use of the antiandrogens (spironolactone, cimetidine, and cyproterone acetate) are helpful. Other cosmetic measures are important to reduce the hirsutism. Techniques to remove the unwanted hair include bleaching, tweezing, hot wax epilation, chemical depilatories, shaving, and electrolysis. <u>Shaving is the safest way to remove hair and has the least untoward reactions</u>. Patients should be informed that shaving does not increase hair growth or increase the thickness of the hair shaft. <u>The only permanent means of removing the hair is to ablate the hair follicle</u>. Electrolysis or short-wave radio frequency

HIRSUTISM 155

thermolysis is effective but requires the skill of an experienced electrologist and is expensive. The combination of medical therapy, frequent shaving, judicious electrolysis, and a sympathetic physician are necessary to successfully manage this common medical problem.

PEARLS:

1. Hair growth is interpreted differently by each patient. Our culture glorifies hairless women (e.g., models found on magazine covers). Important factors for hirsutism include race (Orientals, American Indians, and Negroes have less hirsutism than Caucasians), genetic background (those of Mediterranean origin are typically more hirsute than those of Nordic origin), complexion (darkly pigmented Caucasian women tend to be more hirsute than light-complected females), age (incidence of hirsutism increases after menopause), and family history. Some women complain of relatively mild hirsutism, not realizing the range of normal variation and the significance of the factors mentioned above.

2. In evaluating hirsutism, age of onset and the rapidity of progression are important. Virilizing signs (increased muscle mass, deepening of voice, clitoromelagy, amenorrhea) occurring prior to puberty should lead one to consider congenital adrenal hyperplasia, childhood Cushing's syndrome, or ovarian tumor. Recent onset of progressive hair growth associated with virilizing signs in post-menarche females suggests a serious underlying process (ovarian/adrenal tumor) and should lead to intensive investigation to the cause.

3. Hyperandrogenism causes hirsutism in most patients (> 95%). Testosterone is the primary androgen that stimulates the hair follicle. The testosterone production rate is increased in

156   CASE STUDIES IN ENDOCRINOLOGY

nearly all hirsute women although the serum or plasma testosterone may be in the upper range of normal.

4. Testosterone is produced from three sources in the normal female: ovary (25% of the total), adrenal (25% of the total), and peripheral tissues (50% of the total). The peripheral tissues (fat, muscle) convert weak androgens (primarily androstenedione) secreted by the adrenal and ovary into testosterone. In evaluating the hirsute female, one tries to identify the source of the hyperandrogenemia: ovary, adrenal, or both.

5. Although the serum testosterone level may not accurately reflect the severity of the hyperandrogenic state, persistent testosterone values greater than 200 ng/dl require excluding an ovarian tumor and, though much less likely, an adrenal tumor.

6. Elevated urine 17-ketosteroids suggest an adrenal source. Ketosteroid values are normal or minimally elevated in female with androgenized ovary syndrome (PCOD). DHEA-S is the major precursor of urine 17-ketosteroids. Where urine collections are not easily obtained, serum DHEA-S can be measured.

7. A few hirsute females (often with normal menstruation and very mild hair growth) have a late-onset or adult form of congenital adrenal hyperplasia. In this syndrome (1 to 8% of hirsute women), there is a partial block in 21-hydroxylase activity which leads to elevated serum levels of 17-hydroxyprogesterone (17-OHP). These patients are diagnosed by a provocative ACTH study. Baseline 17-OHP is drawn, and cosyntropin 0.25 mg is administered intramuscularly, and serum 17-OHP is measured 1 hour later. Patients with a partial enzymatic defect demonstrate a 5 to 10-fold rise in 17-OHP levels (normal, less than two-fold

HIRSUTISM 157

rise). Treatment consists of dexamethasone 0.5 mg at bedtime (alternatively, prednisone 5 mg at bedtime).

8. The androgen metabolite <u>androstanediol glucuronide</u> is the most sensitive marker of androgen stimulation at the hair follicle. As mentioned above, DHT is the potent androgen that causes hair growth. DHT is metabolized to androstanediol and androstanediol glucuronide. Levels of the 3-alpha-diol glucuronide in hirsute women are 10-12 times higher than those of normal women. Changes in this metabolite are much more pronounced than serum testosterone levels (including free testosterone) and offer a marker of hirsutism and a potential guide to follow therapy of hirsute women.

PITFALLS:

1. <u>Serum testosterone levels are only indirect determinations of androgen activity.</u> The free or unbound testosterone, the bioactive moiety, constitutes less than 1-3% of the total serum testosterone, the remainder being bound to sex hormone-binding globulin (SHBG). Hyperandrogenemia lowers SHBG levels (decreases hepatic SHBG production) so that the total serum testosterone is a poor reflection of androgen status.

2. A 24-hour urine for 17-ketosteroids reflects the serum DHEA-S and androstenedione concentrations and evaluates <u>adrenal</u> androgen output. 17-Ketosteroids do <u>not</u> measure testosterone.

3. Dynamic studies such as dexamethasone suppression studies and gonadotropin stimulatory studies do <u>not</u> help distinguish whether the androgen source is the adrenal or ovary and are generally avoided.

158 CASE STUDIES IN ENDOCRINOLOGY

4. Even if the source of hyperandrogenemia is removed (e.g., adrenal adenoma or ovarian arrhenoblastoma), one should not be too optimistic regarding eradication of hirsutism. In such cases features of virilization often persist for years. Once the hair follicle in the androgen-sensitive areas is stimulated, only small amounts of androgens are necessary for continued hair growth. With time, however, the rate and amount of hair growth decrease.

REFERENCES

Givens JR: Hirsutism. In Krieger DT, Bardin CW (eds): Current Therapy in Endocrinology 1983-1984. Burlington, Ontario, B.C. Decker, 1983, pp 143-146.

Kirschner MA: Hirsutism and virilization in women. Special Topics in Endocrinology and Metabolism 6:55, 1984.

Kirschner MA, Zucker IR, Jepersen D: Idiopathic hirsutism—an ovarian abnormality. N Engl J Med 294:637, 1976.

Kuttenn F, Couillin P, Girard F, et al: Late-onset adrenal hyperplasia. N Engl J Med 313:224, 1985.

Pehrson JJ, Vaitukaitis J, Longcope C: Bromocriptine, sex steroid metabolism, and menstrual patterns in the polycystic ovarian syndrome. Ann Intern Med 105:129, 1986.

Yen SSC: The polycystic ovary syndrome. Clin Endocrinol 12:177, 1980.

Zumoff B, Freeman R, Coupey S, et al: A chronobiologic abnormality in luteinizing hormone secretion in teenage girls with the polycystic-ovary syndrome. N Engl J Med 309:1206, 1983.

TEENAGER WITH AMENORRHEA

CASE 21: K.K., a 16-year-old high school student, presented for the evaluation of amenorrhea. She developed nipple budding at 11 years of age which progressed over the next 4 years to full breast development. When she was 12 years, pubic and axillary hair growth began. She achieved normal height and weight and was elected "Miss Teen" of her class. However, she never menstruated. The family history was negative for any endocrine disease. She had three younger sisters.

This young woman weighed 119 lb; height, 66 inches; BP, 105/60; pulse, 70/min. She was an attractive female with a clear complexion without acne or hirsutism. The axillae were shaven, but the pubic hair appeared decreased in thickness. The breasts were well developed. There was no galactorrhea. Pelvic exam showed normal female external genitalia without clitoromegaly. Speculum exam of the vagina failed to visualize the cervix. No uterus or adnexal masses were palpable. HEENT, heart, abdominal, and neurological exams were normal.

160　CASE STUDIES IN ENDOCRINOLOGY

ENDOCRINE CLUE: The buccal mucosa was scraped with a tongue blade and the cells were stained.

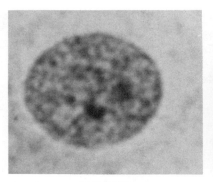 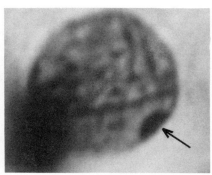

PATIENT　　　　　　　　**FEMALE CONTROL**

QUESTIONS:

1. What diagnoses should you consider in 16-year-old females who have never menstruated?

2. What does the CLUE show and what do these findings mean?

3. What is this patient's diagnosis and what is the nature of this disorder?

4. What laboratory studies should you order on this patient and what would be the expected results?

5. Why is she so well estrogenized?

6. How should she be managed?

7. How would you work up an amenorrheic patient of child-bearing age when the diagnosis is not evident from the history and physical examination?

162   CASE STUDIES IN ENDOCRINOLOGY

ANSWERS:

1. This patient has primary amenorrhea (absence of menses in females < 16 years of age). Causes of primary amenorrhea (listed in order of decreasing frequency) include: **a**) Turner's syndrome (gonadal dysgenesis) with sexual infantilism (absent breast development) and its somatic manifestations (short stature, webbed neck, widely spaced nipples, etc.); **b**) congenital absence of vagina with normal growth and sexual development (breast, pubic and axillary hair, feminine figure); **c**) testicular feminization with blind vaginal pouch, scant pubic hair, inguinal hernia, and often palpable inguinal masses; and **d**) imperforate hymen. This patient did not have galactorrhea with amenorrhea to indicate a pituitary abnormality (possible prolactinoma), nor did she have underlying chronic disease (hepatic and renal failure) or any other endocrine disorders such as thyroid disease (hyperthyroidism and hypothyroidism), adrenal disease (hypocortisolism and hypercortisolism), and hirsutism. A history of weight loss, amenorrhea, bulemia, and bradycardia in a otherwise healthy teenager suggests anorexia nervosa. Finally, pregnancy should be considered (though a unlikely cause of primary amenorrhea).

2. The patient's nuclei fail to show an area of intense staining on the periphery of the nucleus. The "sex chromatin" or "Barr body" found in the normal female was absent in this patient (see CLUE; FEMALE CONTROL). The normal female has the karyotype 46,XX and is sex chromatin positive. This patient's buccal smear is consistent with the XO or XY karyotype. This patient would have either gonadal dysgenesis or male pseudohermaphroditism (male karyotype with female phenotype).

3. Testicular feminization. This patient was a well estrogenized female (full breasts and feminine distribution of body fat)

TEENAGER WITH AMENORRHEA   163

which suggests that functioning gonads were present. In contrast, patients with Turner's syndrome would be estrogen deficient, lacking development of secondary sex features. The blind vaginal pouch, absent uterus, and the sex chromatin negative buccal smear suggest testicular feminization. The buccal smear would be sex chromatin positive in patients with congenital absence of the uterus. This patient has testes that make testosterone but complete androgen resistance causes the female phenotype. The testes *in utero* produce Mullerian inhibitory factor, causing the uterus and oviduct to regress (as it does in normal males). This is an X-linked disorder in which affected genotypic males are phenotypic females.

4. Order serum testosterone, serum LH (luteinizing hormone), and serum estradiol. The level of serum testosterone will be in the male range (300-1000 ng/dl). The serum LH level will be relatively elevated (androgen resistance at the level of hypothalamic-pituitary leads to an increase in LH pulse frequency and amplitude of LH spikes). The serum estradiol will be elevated (for men). Confirming the 46,XY karyotype helps in counseling family members. Remember that this patient has three phenotypic sisters who might have the same diagnosis.

5. Elevated estradiol levels and resistance to androgens make for a very feminine phenotype. The elevated estradiol comes from two sources: **a**) augmented LH secretion that increases testicular production of estradiol, and **b**) increased peripheral conversion of androstenedione and testosterone to estradiol.

6. First, assure the patient of her feminine gender. Educate the patient that her problem is a genetic condition that makes menstruation and fertility impossible. Sonograms will confirm the presence of intra-abdominal testes. As soon as

164   CASE STUDIES IN ENDOCRINOLOGY

puberty is complete, then surgical removal of the testes is recommended to avoid cancerous development of the gonads (incidence of neoplasia approaches 50% in women > 30 years old). After surgery, replacement with estrogen is prescribed to maintain secondary sex characteristics and to avoid hypogonadism. Reconstructive surgery may be necessary if the vaginal pouch is inadequate in length for sexual intercourse.

7. First, rule out pregnancy. If the urine pregnancy test for chorionic gonadotropin (or serum beta-HCG) is negative, the following studies are performed: a) serum prolactin to assess whether hyperprolactinemia is the cause of the secondary amenorrhea; b) serum gonadotropins (FSH and LH) to determine if there is primary ovarian failure; and c) progestin administration to assess the level of endogenous estrogen and the competence of the outlet tract. Medroxyprogesterone acetate (10-mg tablet) is taken daily for 5 days. Vaginal bleeding should occur within a week after the medroxyprogesterone is discontinued. Withdrawal bleeding indicates normal endogenous estrogen levels since proliferative endometrium (which is under estrogenic stimulation) must be present if progesterone is to have an effect (progesterone converts proliferative endometrium into a secretive endometrium). Withdrawal bleeding will not occur in outlet obstruction (congenital absent vagina), uterine agenesis (testicular feminization, XY gonadal dysgenesis), endometrial scarring (Asherman's syndrome), or in the "unprimed" uterus of low estrogen states (gonadal failure, hypopituitarism). Patients who have withdrawal bleeding and normal serum prolactin levels have anovulation as the etiology of their amenorrhea (polycystic ovarian disease, extraglandular estrogen formation, psychogenic causes). An additional study to perform in women who do not have withdrawal bleeding after progestin administration is to prime the endometrium with estrogen (conjugated

estrogens 1.25 mg twice a day for 21 days) followed by progesterone (medroxyprogesterone 10 mg each day for 5 days). Withdrawal bleeding will not occur in <u>outlet obstruction</u> or <u>end-organ abnormality</u> (uterine agenesis or Asherman's syndrome). Females with testicular feminization will not have withdrawal bleeding since no uterus is present.

PEARLS:

1. This paradigm is useful in evaluating patients whose amenorrhea is not certain after the history and physical examination and after pregnancy has been excluded.

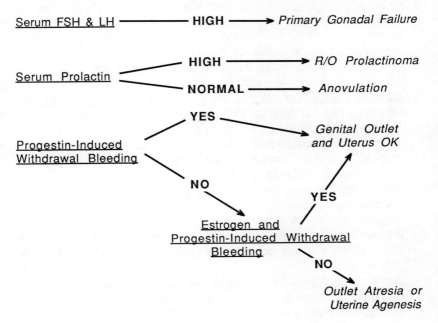

166   CASE STUDIES IN ENDOCRINOLOGY

2. Testicular feminization occurs in about 1 out of 50,000 male births. One famous woman who might have had this syndrome is Queen Elizabeth I.

3. Since the skin and its appendages are not stimulated by normal or high normal levels of serum testosterone in testicular feminization, these patients are often called "hairless women."

4. The gonadotropins, FSH and LH, are elevated in gonadal failure. <u>FSH values > 40 mIU/ml are diagnostic of primary gonadal failure.</u> LH levels are elevated prior to ovulation and are not as specific for gonadal failure as raised FSH levels.

5. <u>Postpartum amenorrhea</u> and the inability to nurse may be secondary to pituitary hemorrhage (Sheehan's syndrome). Amenorrhea due to destruction of the endometrium and scarification as a result of overzealous postpartum curettage (Asherman's syndrome) should also be considered.

6. <u>Turner's syndrome is the most common cause of primary amenorrhea.</u> Patients with typical Turner's syndrome have short stature (rarely > 58 inches), a stocky build, a webbed neck, widely spaced nipples ("shield chest"), and cubitus valgus.   These patients have the 45,XO genotype, but mosaicism is common (XO/XX).   Since mosaicism has such grave implications, a cell surface marker of the masculine gender (H-Y antigen) should be sought if the karyotype is negative for the Y chromosome in patients who do <u>not</u> have the typical features of Turner's syndrome.   Gonadectomy is necessary for those patients with evidence of Y chromosome.

7. An easy schedule for prescribing estrogen replacement is: on days 1 through 24 of each month, take 1.25 mg of conjugated estrogens, and on days 20 through 24, take 10 mg of medroxyprogesterone in addition to the estrogen.

Beginning medication on the first of every month establishes an easily remembered routine. Menstruation usually begins on the 27th day of each month.

PITFALLS:

1. Not every patient with testicular feminization has complete androgen resistance. Incomplete androgen resistance leads to variants that have genital ambiguity and predominantly male phenotype (e.g., Reifenstein's syndrome).

2. The diagnosis of testicular feminization should be suspected at birth or early childhood in any female with an inguinal hernia and a mass in the inguinal region or labia.

3. Any hypergonadotropic patient < 35 years of age with primary amenorrhea needs karyotyping to exclude the presence of Y chromosome since the incidence of malignant tumors developing within dysgenetic gonads is about 25%.

REFERENCES

Bakin R: Queen Elizabeth I: a case of testicular feminization? Med Hypotheses 17:277, 1985.

Bardin CW, Wright W: Androgen receptor deficiency: testicular feminization, its variants, and differential diagnosis. Ann Clin Res 12:236, 1980.

Griffin JE, Wilson JD: Disorders of androgen receptor function. Ann NY Acad Sci 438:61, 1984.

Mashchak CA, Kletzky OA, Davajan V: Clinical and laboratory evaluation of patients with primary amenorrhea. Obstet Gynecol 57:715, 1981.

HYPOGLYCEMIA

CASE 22: S.U., a 34-year-old realtor, presents for the evaluation of low blood sugar. For the past two months she has had episodes of confusion such that she could not remember simple items such as counting money, making grocery lists, or even her children's names. Her family noted that she appeared "in a daze" early in the morning, but she improved considerably after breakfast. During the day she would often munch, something she was not accustomed to doing. Food helped her symptoms of hunger and anxiousness. She had gained 5 lb over this interval. She had read about hypoglycemia in a recent magazine article and wondered whether low blood sugar could be her problem. Past medical history, social history, and family history were unremarkable. She denied use of any medications.

On examination, mental status and neurological exams were normal. No needle puncture sites or subcutaneous ecchymoses were identified. The remainder of her physical exam was normal (weight, 130 lb; height, 64 inches; BP, 125/80; pulse, 70/min).

ENDOCRINE CLUE:

Her physician had ordered a fasting plasma glucose. The level was 46 mg/dl. The patient was asymptomatic at the time, though 30 minutes later, prior to eating breakfast, she became confused.

HYPOGLYCEMIA   169

QUESTIONS:

1. How do you define hypoglycemia?

2. Into what categories may hypoglycemia be grouped clinically?

3. What studies would you recommend for this patient?

4. What is the most likely diagnosis and what further studies would you recommend?

5. Knowing the results of these studies (Answer #4), how would you manage this problem?

170   CASE STUDIES IN ENDOCRINOLOGY

ANSWERS:

1. Hypoglycemia must be defined operationally as a blood glucose low enough to produce neuroglycopenic and/or homeostatic (adrenergic) symptoms. Neuroglycopenia may present as inability to concentrate, confusion, incoherent speech, headache, blurred vision, bizarre behavior, focal or generalized seizures, stupor, coma, and finally death. Homeostatic symptoms relate to the sympathomimetic stimulation of hormones including epinephrine, norepinephrine, cortisol, glucagon, and growth hormone which will raise blood glucose in response to hypoglycemia. These homeostatic responses produce the most striking symptoms, including sweating, palpitations, hunger, tachycardia, tremor, and anxiety.

   A diagnosis of hypoglycemia is made when the patient has the symptoms listed above and plasma glucose levels < 60 mg/dl after overnight fast in both males and females or < 50 mg/dl on an oral glucose tolerance test or < 45 mg/dl for females and < 55 mg/dl for males after a 72-hour fast. Symptoms alone do not make a diagnosis of hypoglycemia since most of these reflect nonspecific increase in adrenergic discharge, nor do low plasma glucose levels alone establish the diagnosis of hypoglycemia unless there are accompanying neuroglycopenic or homeostatic symptoms.

2. Hypoglycemia can be grouped into three major categories: induced, fasting, and postprandial hypoglycemia. Induced or exogenous hypoglycemia is by far the most common and is caused by the administration of medication (insulin, sulfonylureas, salicylates) or ingestion of toxic chemicals (alcohol). Fasting hypoglycemias may be caused by endocrine disease (insulinomas, extra-pancreatic tumors, adrenal insufficiency, pituitary insufficiency), hepatic disorders (glycogen storage disease, deficiency of gluconeogenic

HYPOGLYCEMIA 171

enzymes, acute hepatic necrosis), or, rarely, substrate deficiency in which the liver cannot produce enough glucose from lack of precursors (fasting hypoglycemia of pregnancy, ketotic hypoglycemia of childhood, uremia, and starvation). Postprandial or reactive hypoglycemia is the catch-all category characterized by hypoglycemic symptoms (adrenergic type) that develop with a few hours of eating (idiopathic reactive hypoglycemia, hereditary fructose intolerance).

3. Her symptoms are compatible with hypoglycemia, but low blood sugars need to be documented. Ideally, one would like to get a plasma glucose during and episode or "spell" and correlate the level of glucose with symptoms. Otherwise the time at which the blood is drawn depends on your index of suspicion as to the cause of hypoglycemia. Fasting hypoglycemia is a good possibility for this patient. So you might ask for a fasting plasma glucose with a concomitant insulin level. Alternatively, if a standard oral glucose tolerance test is ordered, the 0 time serves as a fasting level. An oral glucose tolerance test produced the following results:

TIME (hours)	PLASMA GLUCOSE (mg/dl)	PLASMA INSULIN (μU/ml)
0	48	14
1	150	20
2	118	17
3	55	15
4	50	14
5	49	12

4. Fasting hypoglycemia is most likely. Because this condition is associated with significant pathology, the workup should be complete and the diagnosis definitive. By definition, these

172   CASE STUDIES IN ENDOCRINOLOGY

patients fail to maintain plasma glucose homeostasis when food is withheld. <u>You should order a 72-hour fast with plasma glucoses and insulins drawn every 6 hours or until symptoms develop</u>. Hyperinsulinism secondary to insulin-producing pancreatic islet adenoma (insulinoma) is diagnosed when the fasting plasma glucose is low (< 45 mg/dl) and the plasma insulin level is inappropriately elevated (> 6 µU/ml). Twelve hours into a 72-hour fast, this patient became sweaty, confused, and glassy-eyed. The plasma glucose was 39 mg/dl and the insulin level was 12 µU/ml. This confirms hyperinsulinism. Once this diagnosis is made, the site of insulin overproduction must be determined. <u>Order abdominal CT scan</u>. *[CT was reported as normal.]* <u>Order selective mesenteric arteriography</u>. *[The arteriogram showed a questionable "blush" in the mid-pancreas.]* Selective venous sampling of the portal system looking for gradients in insulin levels helps to localize the tumor.

5. Since an insulinoma is likely, <u>surgical removal of the tumor is the treatment of choice</u>. Uncertainty always lingers concerning the diagnosis and treatment of insulinoma. For example, the Mayo Clinic series reported 5.4% operative mortality in 154 patients treated for insulinoma. In over 10% of the cases the tumor was not found at surgery. Although selective mesenteric arteriography can help locate the tumor, the surgeon's skill and expertise are really the most critical factors in identifying and removing these tumors. <u>Diazoxide</u> may be tried in patients who refuse surgery or those whose hyperinsulinism is not cured by surgery. Metastatic islet cell tumors do respond to streptozocin, but the response is unfortunately not curative.

HYPOGLYCEMIA 173

PEARLS:

1. Several factors (gender, antecedent level of glucose, and rapidity of fall) determine whether a particular level of glucose will produce symptoms. Healthy females have a 10-15 mg/dl lower plasma glucose level than males during a 72-hour fast. The antecedent level of plasma glucose is also important since diabetic patients with chronic hyperglycemia may manifest hypoglycemic symptoms at plasma glucose 90-100 mg/dl, whereas normal subjects with glucose levels raised acutely to 300 mg/dl and then reduced abruptly will not have any symptoms until the plasma glucose is reduced to < 50 mg/dl. The rapidity of the plasma glucose fall may determine whether symptoms will occur, but again the level of blood/plasma glucose itself is the most critical parameter for whether symptoms develop.

2. The fragment that binds the A and B chains of proinsulin (connecting peptide or C-peptide) is secreted in amounts equimolar to insulin. Assaying for C-peptide is helpful in factitious insulin abuse where the level will be low, but such an assay is not helpful in sulfonylurea abuse where the levels will be high. Urinary screening for sulfonylureas should be positive in these instances. Obtaining blood levels of chlorpropamide is also helpful.

3. Mesothelial-derived tumors (retroperitoneal fibrosarcomas, hemangiopericytomas), hepatomas, and adrenal carcinomas may present with fasting hypoglycemia. These tumors are large and generally easily palpable as abdominal masses. The mechanism by which the tumors cause hypoglycemia is unknown. Insulin levels are low. In some patients (40%) radioimmunoassayable insulin-like growth factor (IGF) is elevated. The tumor may overutilize glucose because of sheer bulk, but most likely some product is released which inhibits hepatic gluconeogenesis/glycogenolysis.

174   CASE STUDIES IN ENDOCRINOLOGY

4. <u>Alcohol-induced   hypoglycemia</u> is typically seen in binge drinkers or in malnourished individuals.   Hypoglycemia develops 6-24 hours after drinking ceases.   These patients present with hypothermia, coma, plasma glucoses (< 30 mg/dl), tachypnea (lactic acidosis), with or without ethanol on the breath, blood ethanol levels below those of acute intoxication, and abnormal liver function studies.   Patients with   alcohol-induced   hypoglycemia   do   <u>not</u> have a hyperglycemic response to intramuscular glucagon since their livers are depleted of glycogen.

PITFALLS:

1. <u>The most common fasting hypoglycemia is factitious</u>. These patients have plasma glucoses as low and insulins as high as those patients with insulinoma.   They surreptitiously inject insulin or ingest oral hypoglycemic agents and present for management of fasting hypoglycemia even though they really fall into the induced hypoglycemia category.   Paramedical individuals (nurses, pharmacists, etc.) or relatives of diabetic patients are suspect for this problem.

2. A properly performed fast is difficult to obtain. Invariably the patient will receive orange juice for a "spell" or for low readings on a reflectometer without any symptoms.   Do not trust the reflectometer for low readings. <u>Always make sure that the patient has a plasma glucose and insulin drawn prior to aborting the fast</u>.   Let your covering physician know that a fast is in progress, so when he or she gets the 2 AM phone call that Ms. Smith has a Dextrostix® reading of 39, he/she will know what to do.

HYPOGLYCEMIA 175

3. <u>Induced hypoglycemias</u> do not require an exhausting workup, but a carefully taken history is mandatory. Is the diabetic taking too much insulin? Is the diabetic runner or bicyclist injecting the leg instead of the abdomen? (Insulin absorption is better in an exercising limb.) Is the insulin injected intramuscularly versus subcutaneously? (Intramuscular injections are likely to be rapidly absorbed, leading to possible hypoglycemia.)

4. <u>Idiopathic or reactive hypoglycemia</u> can be diagnosed when the symptoms of hypoglycemia are associated temporally with plasma glucose < 50 mg/dl after a meal. The nadir occurs between 3 and 4 hours after feeding, with a return to normal fasting values by the 5th and 6th hours. If there is no rebound to normal values (as the case presented above), then a workup to exclude fasting hypoglycemia (insulinoma, adrenal or pituitary insufficiency) should be considered.

5. Many patients make their own diagnosis of <u>reactive hypoglycemia</u>, attributing the symptoms of adrenergic discharge, mental and physical fatigue, and weakness that may or may not be relieved by glucose-laden food or beverages to "hypoglycemia." Unfortunately, there is not a study that can mimic the conditions under which these patients have symptoms. The time-honored oral glucose tolerance test (GTT) has its problems. Most patients being evaluated for hypoglycemia with the GTT have symptoms when the corresponding plasma glucoses are in the normal range.

6. Most patients who have low plasma glucoses at 2-4 hours during the GTT do not have decreased plasma glucose following a <u>normal</u> meal. Low plasma glucoses cannot be definitively related to symptoms in more than 95% of patients in whom the diagnosis of reactive hypoglycemia is tentatively made.

176   CASE STUDIES IN ENDOCRINOLOGY

REFERENCES

Burch WM: Hypoglycemia: a handle that rarely fits. NC Med J 45:765, 1984.

Charles MA, Hofeldt F, Shackelford A, et al: Comparison of oral glucose tolerance tests and mixed meals in patients with apparent idiopathic postabsorptive hypoglycemia: absence of hypoglycemia after meals. Diabetes 30:465, 1981.

Ensinck JW: Postprandial hypoglycemia. In Kreiger DT, Bardin CW (eds): Current Therapy in Endocrinology 1983-1984. Burlington, Ontario, B.C. Decker, 1983, pp 215-222.

Hogan MJ, Service FJ, Sharbrough FW, Gerich JE: Oral glucose tolerance test compared with a mixed meal in the diagnosis of reactive hypoglycemia: a caveat on stimulation. Mayo Clin Proc 58:491, 1983.

Johnson DD, Dorr KE, Swenson WM, Service J: Reactive hypoglycemia. JAMA 243:1151, 1980.

Lev-Ran A, Anderson RW: The diagnosis of postprandial hypoglycemia. Diabetes 30:996, 1981.

Nelson RL: Hypoglycemia: fact or fiction? Mayo Clin Proc 60:844, 1985.

Sherwin RS, Felig P: Hypoglycemia. In Felig P, Baxter JD, Broadus AE, Frohman LA (eds): Endocrinology and Metabolism. New York, McGraw-Hill, 1981, pp 869-889.

WEAKNESS AND "DRAWING" OF THE HANDS

CASE 23: T.I., a 65-year-old widow, presented with the chief complaint of weakness. She had been walking to her mailbox (100 feet) daily, but for the last week she had difficulty getting out of bed because of lower extremity weakness. She was carried to the emergency room where you see her. She denied any loss of consciousness, bowel or bladder difficulty, or pain the lower extremities. She had intermittent leg cramps and occasional "drawing" of the hands. The medical history was significant. She had had diabetes mellitus for 16 years and was taking a single daily injection of insulin (NPH 20 U each AM). She had very infrequent hypoglycemic episodes. Complications of diabetes included proliferative retinopathy OD treated with photocoagulation (visual acuity OU, 20/50) and relatively asymptomatic peripheral neuropathy (nocturnal foot pain relieved with two aspirin tablets). Fourteen years ago, she had a bleeding peptic ulcer that was treated by a Billroth II gastrectomy. There had been no recurrence of this problem. She lived alone in a trailer park.

Physical examination revealed a chronically ill woman who weighed 105 lb; height, 62 inches; BP, 130/90; pulse, 90/min and regular; temperature, 98.7°F. The skin was pale with senile purpura over the dorsal forearms. The eye exam revealed photocoagulation scars and background retinopathy. Cataracts were not present. She was edentulous. No thyromegaly was noted. Chest and heart exams were normal. A midline abdominal scar above the umbilicus was normally pigmented and well healed. Neurological exam showed normal mental status, but poor strength in the upper and lower extremities. Both thighs showed wasting. She could stand with assistance but could not arise from a squatting position. No fasciculations were observed. Sensory exam showed decreased pinprick and vibratory sensation up to both knees. Knee and ankle reflexes were absent.

178   CASE STUDIES IN ENDOCRINOLOGY

ENDOCRINE CLUE: The following laboratory studies were obtained: Hemoglobin, 11.2 gm; hemocrit, 33.4%; mean corpuscular volume, 102. Urine analysis: no glucose; 1+ protein; no cells. <u>Serum:</u> BUN, 20 mg/dl; creatinine, 1.1 mg/dl; glucose, 150 mg/dl; K, 4.2 mEq/l; calcium, 6.5 mg/dl; phosphate, 2.7 mg/dl; total protein, 5.9 gm/dl; albumin, 3.0 gm/dl; alkaline phosphatase, 310 U/l (normal, 30-110).

WEAKNESS AND "DRAWING" OF THE HANDS   179

QUESTIONS:

1. What physical findings should you go back and look for in this patient?

2. What are the possible causes of hypocalcemia?

3. What is the most likely cause of the hypocalcemia?

4. What studies might you order to confirm this diagnosis?

5. How would you manage this patient's problems?

180   CASE STUDIES IN ENDOCRINOLOGY

ANSWERS:

1. The physical exam was nearly complete, but the finding of hypocalcemia should make you return to the bedside and check for signs of latent tetany. Look for Trousseau's sign (inflate the sphygmomanometer 20 mm above systolic pressure for 3 minutes and observe for carpal spasm and thenar adduction: flexion of the wrist and metacarpophalangeal joints and adduction of the thumb) and Chvostek's sign (tapping the facial nerve over the parotid elicits a twitch at the angle of the mouth). *[Trousseau's and Chvostek's signs were elicited in this patient.]*

2. The differential diagnosis of hypocalcemia includes: hypomagnesemia; hypoparathyroidism due to parathyroid hormone (PTH) deficiency or resistance (pseudohypoparathyroidism); pancreatitis; acute phosphate intoxication; and vitamin D deficiency (e.g., malabsorption) and disorders of vitamin D metabolism (e.g., renal insufficiency). Hypoalbuminemia might also be added the the list (the serum calcium will be low, but the ionized calcium will be normal). You ought to exclude hypomagnesemia as a cause of hypocalcemia; order serum Mg. *[Mg level returns at 1.9 mEq/l--normal.]* Hypoparathyroidism is unlikely because the serum phosphorus is not elevated.

3. Vitamin D deficiency is most likely in this patient. Several factors point to this diagnosis: **a**) calcium intake in elderly women is historically low and sun exposure often limited; **b**) patients with gastrectomy, particularly with Billroth II anastomoses, may malabsorb calcium and vitamin D; and **c**) other causes of hypocalcemia seem unlikely. Patients with hypoparathyroidism often have higher levels of serum phosphorus. Vitamin D deficiency or altered vitamin D metabolism leads to inadequate calcium absorption from the gut and low serum calcium. Secondary hyperparathyroidism

WEAKNESS AND "DRAWING" OF THE HANDS   181

results from the attempt to normalize serum calcium and leads to lowering of the serum phosphorus as a result of PTH-induced phosphaturia. Serum alkaline phosphatase activity is elevated by osteoblastic activation coupled to bone resorption effects of PTH. The serum chemistries in this patient suggest secondary hyperparathyroidism (low serum P) and increased bone turnover (raised serum alkaline phosphatase) found in vitamin D deficiency and osteomalacia. The elevated MCV (> 100) again suggests a malabsorption problem (folate deficiency or low vitamin B12 level). She may have blind loop syndrome due to Billroth II anastomoses leading to malabsorption.

4. <u>Order serum 25-hydroxyvitamin D</u>. The level of serum 25-hydroxyvitamin D, which is the best indicator of body stores of vitamin D, is low when vitamin D is deficient. *[Serum 25-OHD was 7 ng/ml (normal, 15 to 80).]* <u>Order serum folate and B12 levels</u>. *[Serum folate is normal, but B12 level is borderline low.]* <u>Bone marrow</u> shows no Fe and mild megaloblastic changes. <u>Order serum PTH level</u>. In vitamin D deficiency, PTH levels are extremely high. As expected, the serum PTH in this patient was elevated (12.5 ng/ml; normal, 0.4-1.5). A bone biopsy was obtained and showed osteomalacia. A small bowel biopsy showed no villous atrophy.

5. <u>This woman needs calcium supplementation and vitamin D or one of its analogs for treatment of chronic hypocalcemia.</u> Doses in the range of 1.5-2.5 gm of elemental calcium per day are prescribed in divided doses three times a day. The calcium content of the available preparations varies, and one must be certain that the proper amount of elemental calcium is given. Calcium carbonate is the most convenient form since the high calcium content (40%) of this compound means fewer tablets are needed. Calcium chloride should be avoided because of the high incidence of gastric irritation.

182 CASE STUDIES IN ENDOCRINOLOGY

CALCIUM PREPARATIONS USED IN TREATING CHRONIC HYPOCALCEMIA

COMPOUND	TRADE NAME	CALCIUM CONTENT	TABS/DAY	COST/DAY
Calcium Carbonate	Generic 500	500 mg	3	$.07-.10
	OsCal 500	500 mg	3	$.40-.50
	Titralac 420 mg	168 mg	9	$.55-.75
	Tums	200 mg	8	$.30-.40
Calcium Lactate	Generic 625 mg	80 mg	19	$.50-.75
Calcium Gluconate	Generic 1 gm	90 mg	17	$1.60
Calcium Glubionate	Neo-Calglucon 5 ml	115 mg	4 tbsp	$1.85

This table lists several calcium preparations, their calcium content, and the approximate cost per day to the patient for 1.5 gm of elemental calcium.

Vitamin D-related osteomalacia is usually treated with vitamin D2, the plant-derived vitamin, which is inexpensive. Each vitamin D preparation has its advantages and its disadvantages. D2 is cheap and usually effective, but the therapeutic dose approaches the toxic dose, the onset of action is slow (weeks), and the duration is prolonged since this vitamin is stored in fat. Pharmacological doses up to 100,000 IU of D2/day are required to treat osteomalacia due to bowel malabsorption (D2 may need to be administered intramuscularly if oral D2 fails). Other preparations are available (25-hydroxyvitamin D and dihydrotachysterol) but these are relatively expensive and offer no real practical advantages. Calcitriol (1,25-dihydroxyvitamin D) is expensive ($60-70 per 100 0.25-μg tabs), but its onset of action is rapid (2-4 days) and its half-life is short (12 hours).

WEAKNESS AND "DRAWING" OF THE HANDS   183

In addition to calcium and vitamin D supplementation, oral ferrous sulfate and monthly B12 injections were prescribed for this patient.

PEARLS:

1. The severity and duration of the hypocalcemia dictates the clinical presentation. Acute hypocalcemia is much more likely to be symptomatic than chronic hypocalcemia despite equivalent levels of serum calcium. Signs and symptoms of neuromuscular irritability predominate and include weakness, muscle cramps, paresthesias of the hands and feet, and tetany. Epileptiform seizures and laryngospasm are common presentations in children.

2. Cataracts may form in chronic hypocalcemia. The cause is unknown, but correction of the hypocalcemia halts further progression.

3. Since about half of the total serum calcium is bound to protein, a low serum calcium should be anticipated in cases of hypoalbuminemia. As a rule, for each gram of albumin below 4 gm/dl, the total serum calcium should be lowered by 0.8 mg/dl. Thus, the "corrected" serum Ca in this patient would be 7.3 mg/dl (still a hypocalcemic value). Similarly, albumin levels above 4.0 gm/dl raise serum Ca 0.8 mg/dl for each gram of albumin.

4. Acute hyperventilation leads to alkalosis, which lowers the ionized calcium without changing the total serum calcium.

5. Patients with gluten enteropathy may resolve their osteomalacia with a gluten-free diet alone.

184   CASE STUDIES IN ENDOCRINOLOGY

6. Patients taking anticonvulsant therapy need 5000 IU of D2/day to treat and prevent osteomalacia.

7. Patients with chronic renal failure and vitamin D-resistant rickets type I respond to physiologic amounts of 1,25-dihydroxyvitamin D (0.5-2.0 µg/day).

8. <u>Surgical hypoparathyroidism is the most common cause of hypoparathyroidism.</u> The management of surgical hypoparathyroidism is generally much easier than that of idiopathic hypoparathyroidism since smaller doses of vitamin D or even calcium supplements alone corrects the hypocalcemia, presumably because some PTH is still being produced.

9. Most patients with vitamin D deficiency are hypocalcemic, but the most common cause of rickets in the United States, is X-linked hypophosphatemic vitamin D-resistant rickets, in which the serum calcium is normal. The serum phosphorus is low in this disorder because of renal wasting of phosphorus ("phosphate diabetes").

PITFALLS:

1. Tetany is not specific for hypocalcemia and may be seen in hypomagnesemia, hypokalemia, and respiratory alkalosis (e.g., hyperventilation).

2. A faint Chvostek's sign is present in about 10% of the normal population, but development of a strong Chvostek's sign after neck surgery suggests hypocalcemia. Trousseau's sign is a more reliable indicator of hypocalcemia.

WEAKNESS AND "DRAWING" OF THE HANDS 185

3. Patients treated with vitamin D preparations need to be followed closely to avoid hypercalcemia (vitamin D intoxication).

4. Hypocalcemia after surgery for hyperparathyroidism is usually related to the "hungry bone syndrome." These patients have hypophosphatemia as opposed to the typical hyperphosphatemia of true parathyroid deficiency.

REFERENCES

Audran M, Kumar R: The physiology and pathophysiology of vitamin D. Mayo Clin Proc 60:851, 1985.

Breslau NA, Pak CYC: Hypoparathyroidism. Metabolism 28:1261, 1979.

Broadus AE: Mineral metabolism. In Felig P, Baxter JD, Broadus AE, Frohman LA (eds): Endocrinology and Metabolism. New York, McGraw-Hill, 1981, pp 963-1079.

Garrick R, Ireland AW, Posen S: Bone abnormalities after gastric surgery: a prospective histological study. Ann Intern Med 75:221, 1971.

Imawari M, Kozawa K, Akanuma Y, et al: Serum 25-hydroxyvitamin D and vitamin D-binding protein levels and mineral metabolism after partial and total gastrectomy. Gastroenterology 79:255, 1980.

Nordin BEC, Horsman A, Marshall DH, et al: Calcium requirement and calcium therapy. Clin Orthop 140:216, 1979.

ASYMPTOMATIC HYPERCALCEMIA

CASE 24: E.C., a 54-year-old part-time nurse, came for a routine evaluation and refill of her prescription. Her general health had been excellent except for hypertension noted 10 years ago. The blood pressure had been well controlled on hydrochlorothiazide 25 mg/day. She complained of fatigue and tiredness that seem more than she expected; however, she had been taking care of her grandchildren (ages 4 and 6 years) 5 days a week. She was taking vitamin pills obtained from a local health food store without relief of her symptoms. She continued to have monthly menses and denied any pain, weight loss, dyspnea, cramps, or myalgias.

She weighed 128 lb; height, 64 inches; pulse, 80 and regular; BP 125/85. Her exam was entirely normal except for the finding noted in the CLUE.

ENDOCRINE CLUE:

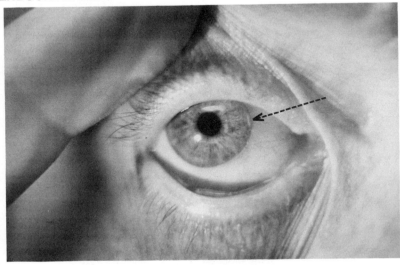

QUESTIONS:

1. What does the CLUE demonstrate and what does it mean?

2. You order a battery of serum chemistries that demonstrate the serum calcium to be 11.1 mg/dl. Other laboratory data include: albumin, 4.0 gm/dl; P, 3.0 mg/dl; BUN, 15 mg/dl; creatinine, 1.0 mg/dl; T4(RIA), 9 µg/dl. What symptoms can you attribute to the hypercalcemia?

3. What are the potential causes of hypercalcemia?

4. What would you recommend next?

5. After reviewing the data obtained in Question #4, what is the most likely diagnosis?

6. What are some of the common problems associated with this diagnosis?

7. How would you manage this problem?

8. In what circumstances would medical therapy be indicated in treating hypercalcemia? What medications could be used?

188 CASE STUDIES IN ENDOCRINOLOGY

ANSWERS:

1. The CLUE shows early <u>band keratopathy</u> (*arrow* points to white line). Band keratopathy commonly begins in the medial and lateral margins of the cornea adjacent to the scleral limbus. The deposition of calcium may extend across the entire cornea as a strip or band. Finding band keratopathy means metastatic calcification and suggests chronic hypercalcemia.

2. <u>Symptoms of hypercalcemia are not specific and are related to the degree and duration of the hypercalcemia.</u> Patients with serum calciums < 11.0 mg/dl are rarely symptomatic with regard to calcium itself, although they may be very symptomatic related to the underlying disease (e.g., malignancy). Levels of serum calcium between 11.0 and 14.0 mg/dl may or may not be associated with symptoms. Hypercalcemia above 14.0 mg/dl is invariably associated with symptoms, and the risk of developing severe organ damage is significant at these levels. General symptoms of weakness, fatigue, and impaired mental concentration are frequent. Polyuria is often observed, but you must ask specifically about voiding habits. Neurologic symptoms include poor recent memory, depression, muscle weakness, and lethargy that can progress to stupor and coma. Gastrointestinal complaints include anorexia, nausea, vomiting, and constipation.

3. Hypercalcemia has multiple etiologies. <u>More than 90% of patients have either primary hyperparathyroidism or malignancy as the cause of hypercalcemia.</u> Other causes are listed in the table on the next page. After reviewing the table, you note that this patient has been on thiazide diuretics and that she may have taken extra quantities of vitamin A or D.

Causes of Hypercalcemia

Primary hyperparathyroidism
  Sporadic (90-95% of the cases of hyperparathyroidism)
  Familial syndromes (MEN I and MEN IIa)
    MEN I (tumors of pituitary, pancreas, and parathyroid)
    MEN IIa (medullary thyroid carcinoma, hyperparathyroidism,
      pheochromocytoma)

Neoplastic diseases
  Local osteolysis (breast and lung carcinoma metastatic
              to bone and myeloma)
  Humoral hypercalcemia of malignancy

Endocrine disorders
  Hyperthyroidism
  Adrenal insufficiency
  Familial hypocalciuric hypercalcemia

Medications
  Thiazide diuretics
  Vitamin D and rarely vitamin A intoxication
  Milk-alkali syndrome
  Phosphodiesterase inhibitors (e.g., theophylline)
  Lithium

Granulomatous diseases
  Sarcoidosis
  Beryllosis, tuberculosis, coccidioidomycosis

Miscellaneous
  Immobilization (associated with high bone turnover rates
              such as in children or patients with Paget's disease)
  Recovery phase of acute renal failure (rare)
  Idiopathic hypercalcemia of infancy (rare)
  Dehydration

190   CASE STUDIES IN ENDOCRINOLOGY

4. First, <u>repeat the serum calcium determination</u>. Although the accuracy is good, bogus values need to be excluded. Calcium is generally measured with colorimetric assays, but atomic absorption and ionized calciums are likely to be more precise. In this case, the band keratopathy pointed to chronic hypercalcemia. *[Repeat serum Ca: 10.9 mg/dl.]* Go over the possible causes of hypercalcemia, then exclude each one as far as possible with history and physical examination and appropriate studies.

    a) Primary hyperparathyroidism. <u>Cannot rule out</u>; <u>order serum PTH</u>; repeat calcium in 2-3 months if other possible causes are excluded.

    b) Neoplastic diseases. Doesn't seem likely in this patient; <u>go back and repeat breast exam</u>. *[Nothing suspicious.]*

    c) Endocrine disorders. No evidence for hyperthyroidism, adrenal insufficiency, or family history of hypercalcemia.

    d) Medications. Maybe; ask specifically about vitamin intake. *[Taking only B complex vitamins.]*
    <u>Discontinue the diuretic for at least 4 weeks</u>, and repeat serum calcium. *[Ca, 11.0 mg/dl 6 weeks later.]*

    e) Granulomatous diseases. Unlikely; no history of sarcoidosis but <u>order a chest X-ray</u> (double check on neoplastic disease as well). *[Chest X-ray, normal.]* In addition, you ask about occupational exposure to beryllium.

<u>You decide to wait for the PTH level to return (takes 1-3 weeks) before making any specific diagnosis</u>. *[PTH level was slightly above the "normal" range and certainly inappropriate for the serum calcium level.]*

5. <u>Primary hyperparathyroidism.</u> This is often a diagnosis of exclusion. Once other causes are thoroughly sought and not found, then primary hyperparathyroidism is most likely. If elevated, the serum PTH helps, but it is not diagnostic.

ASYMPTOMATIC HYPERCALCEMIA 191

6. Prior to the introduction of screening serum profiles, clinical clues to hyperparathyroidism related to <u>renal stones and nephrolithiasis</u> (64% of the cases), <u>bone disease such as osteitis fibrosa cystica</u> (20% of the cases), <u>peptic ulcer disease</u> (12% of the cases), or <u>hypertension</u> (6% of the cases). <u>Pancreatitis</u> is associated with hypercalcemia as are <u>gout</u> and <u>pseudogout</u>. These complications of parathyroid hormone excess are still seen, but the frequency of each has changed because patients are identified before such manifestations are evident.

7. <u>Surgical removal of the parathyroid adenoma or hyperplastic parathyroid glands is the only effective therapy for hyperparathyroidism</u>. The presence of <u>severe hypercalcemia, renal disease, renal stones, bone pain, peptic ulcer, and hypertension</u> are indications for neck exploration. Likewise, patients with MEN I and IIa who have hypercalcemia should have parathyroidectomy. Although the natural history for asymptomatic patients with lesser degrees of hypercalcemia (< 12 mg/dl) is unknown, at least 25% of these patients will have developed some complication attributable to hyperparathyroidism (e.g., decreased creatinine clearance, renal stone, nephrocalcinosis, hypertension, etc.) within 5 years of follow-up. Unfortunately, there is no marker to define which patients will develop complications related to hypercalcemia. <u>The critical factor in the management of the hyperparathyroidism is the availability of an experienced parathyroid surgeon.</u> In most centers, such a surgeon is available, and thus neck exploration is routinely advised even in asymptomatic patients. The surgery is delicate but relatively benign. Most patients are discharged cured on the second or third postoperative day. Advanced age itself is not a contraindication to surgery.

192 CASE STUDIES IN ENDOCRINOLOGY

8. There is no satisfactory medical therapy for primary hyperparathyroidism. However, medical therapy is used in two well-defined areas: life-threatening hypercalcemia and patients who are unacceptable surgical risks. These patients are managed medically with hydration and agents that will acutely lower the serum calcium. Many of these patients have no symptoms directly related to hypercalcemia as long as adequate hydration is assured. Oral phosphates given initially in small doses to avoid diarrhea and increased to 1-2 gm four times a day are reasonable agents to use in an attempt to lower the serum calcium. Careful monitoring of renal function, serum potassium, and serum phosphorus (maintained below 5 mg/dl to minimize ectopic calcification) is necessary. Estrogen (conjugated estrogen 0.625-1.25 mg/day) may be used since estrogen is known to inhibit PTH-induced bone resorption. Despite these measures, there is no ideal therapy for these hypercalcemic patients, who often have underlying illnesses such as hypertension or congestive heart failure which complicate therapy with salt loading and digitalis.

PEARLS:

1. Band keratopathy, a manifestation of metastatic calcification, is a rare but specific sign of chronic hypercalcemia.

2. The deposition of arcus senilis begins superiorly and inferiorly and extends around the margins of the cornea, giving the arcus circularis or anulus senilis. (Remember, band keratopathy starts medially and laterally.) The arcus circularis is separated from the limbus by a clear space within the cornea. This space is often obliterated and filled with whitish deposits in band keratopathy.

ASYMPTOMATIC HYPERCALCEMIA   193

3. Polyuria is an early manifestation of hypercalcemia. Hypercalcemia increases medullary blood flow and washout of gradient and impairs the ability of the renal tubules to respond to vasopressin (ADH) so that urine cannot be maximally concentrated.

4. Patients with hyperparathyroidism generally are asymptomatic and have had the hypercalcemia for sometime prior to the problem being identified. <u>Obtaining old records and reviewing lab studies is well worth the time</u>.

5. A history of hypercalcemia for over a year in the absence of weight loss and other systemic symptoms excludes the other major cause of hypercalcemia (neoplastic disease) and in the absence of other findings (e.g., medications, sarcoidosis) seals the diagnosis of primary hyperparathyroidism.

6. Like many endocrine diseases, hyperparathyroidism is more prevalent in women (from two to five females for every male).

7. Biochemical studies that are helpful but not diagnostic in making the diagnosis of primary hyperparathyroidism include hypophosphatemia (< 3.0 mg/dl), serum chloride > 106 mEq/l, serum chloride/serum phosphorus ratio > 33, elevated serum alkaline phosphatase, or a calcium-phosphate renal stone. Radiographic findings are rare in the asymptomatic patient, but subperiosteal resorption of the phalanges and metacarpals is virtually pathognomonic of hyperparathyroidism.

8. Serum calciums > 14 mg/dl, palpable neck mass, and very high levels of PTH in a patient suspected of hyperparathyroidism should raise the question of <u>parathyroid carcinoma</u>, a rare cause (1-3% of cases) of hyperparathyroidism. Recognition of parathyroid carcinoma is important for surgical cure. *En*

194 CASE STUDIES IN ENDOCRINOLOGY

block resection of tumor and all adjacent invaded tissues (avoiding capsular violation or tumor spillage) is necessary for cure.

9. <u>Vitamin A intoxication</u> may occur with doses > 50,000 U/day. Pharmacologic doses of vitamin A cause osteoclastic bone resorption. Any patient with a skin disorder may be receiving vitamin A; obtaining a good history is important.

10. Recurrence of hyperparathyroidism following parathyroid surgery is most likely in the patients with parathyroid hyperplasia (often the familial syndromes associated with hypercalcemia).

11. Hypercalcemia secondary to primary hyperparathyroidism may be found in each of the familial endocrine neoplasias (MEN) except MEN IIb (pages 75-78). The hyperparathyroidism is usually due to parathyroid hyperplasia in these syndromes.

PITFALLS:

1. Measurement of serum PTH by radioimmunoassay (RIA) may be helpful in questionable cases of hypercalcemia. The RIA for PTH should not be considered as having the same validity as an RIA for growth hormone in acromegaly or insulin in the evaluation of hypoglycemia.

2. Band keratopathy is not specific for hyperparathyroidism and may be found in any condition causing chronic hypercalcemia.

3. Hypocalcemia is the major problem following surgery for hyperparathyroidism in the patient who has <u>bone disease and elevated serum alkaline phosphatase preoperatively.</u> Such

ASYMPTOMATIC HYPERCALCEMIA   195

patients will generally need large doses of calcium intravenously, oral calcium supplements, and possibly short-acting calcitriol (0.5-1.0 µg twice a day) for several weeks postoperatively. By then the "hungry bones" will have reached a state of equilibrium after escaping the resorptive effects of chronic hyperparathyroidism, and the serum alkaline phosphatase and serum phosphorus will have returned to normal. Calcium supplementation can be discontinued. A few patients will have permanent hypoparathyroidism and need indefinite treatment.

4. <u>The patient with hypercalcemia needs to know the importance of good hydration and adequate fluid intake</u>. Dehydration that might lead to hypercalcemic crisis is a major complication in patients with hypercalcemia. If illness intervenes (e.g., viral gastroenteritis), the patient must be warned to get medical attention.

5. Patients who have persistent hypercalcemia after parathyroid surgery for hypercalcemia or positive family history of hypercalcemia should be screened for <u>familial hypocalciuric hypercalcemia</u>. This entity is distinct from primary hyperparathyroidism in several respects: <u>age</u> (a familial disorder in which most patients will be < 20 years of age); <u>urine calcium</u> (urine calcium excretion is inappropriately low for the degree of hypercalcemia, often less than 100 mg/day. Most hyperparathyroid patients excrete > 250 mg/day); <u>complications</u> (nephrolithiasis and peptic ulcer disease are rare); and <u>response to surgery</u> (subtotal parathyroidectomy does not cure the hypercalcemia, although total parathyroidectomy does lead to hypocalcemia). The management of this autosomal dominant syndrome is first "do no harm." Since complications are rare and surgery does not correct the hypercalcemia, operation is avoided.

196 CASE STUDIES IN ENDOCRINOLOGY

REFERENCES

Arnaud CD, Clark OH: Primary hyperparathyroidism. In Krieger DT, Bardin CW (eds): Current Therapy in Endocrinology 1983-1984. Burlington, Ontario, B.C. Decker, 1983, pp 277-282.

Broadus AE: Mineral metabolism,. In Felig P, Baxter JD, Broadus AE, Frohman LA (eds): Endocrinology and Metabolism. New York, McGraw-Hill, 1981, pp 963-1079.

Habener JF, Potts JT: Parathyroid physiology and primary hyperparathyroidism. In Avioli LV, Krane SM (eds): Metabolic Bone Disease, vol 2. New York, Academic Press, 1978, pp 1-147.

Marx SJ, Speigel AM, Brown EM, et al: Divalent cation metabolism. Familial hypocalciuric hypercalcemia versus typical primary hyperparathyroidism. Am J Med 65:235, 1978.

McPherson ML, Prince SR, Atamer ER, et al: Theophylline-induced hypercalcemia. Ann Intern Med 105:52, 1986.

Tibblin S, Palsson N, Rydberg J: Hyperparathyroidism in the elderly. Ann Surg 197:135, 1983.

Wang C, Gaz RD: Natural history of parathyroid carcinoma: diagnosis treatment, and results. Am J Surg 149:522, 1985.

SUDDEN-ONSET BACK PAIN

CASE 25: B.T., a 62-year-old white female, presented with mild back pain. While lifting her 30-lb grandson, she experienced sharp and severe pain in the center of her back between her shoulder blades. The severity of the pain gradually decreased over the following 2 days. Her general health had been excellent. She was taking no medication. Her menses stopped at the age of 55. She smoked one pack of cigarettes daily and drank 2 ounces of gin each evening. There was no history of surgery or family history of endocrine disease.

She weighed 105 lb (height, 63 inches). BP was 110/70; pulse, 78/min. Other than mild thoracic kyphosis and tenderness to hammer percussion over the spinal process of T7-T9, the examination was normal.

198 CASE STUDIES IN ENDOCRINOLOGY

ENDOCRINE CLUE:

Asking about height is helpful; a loss of stature suggests decreased bone mass and means further evaluation is necessary. *[Her former height was 64 inches.]* A lateral chest X-ray was taken.

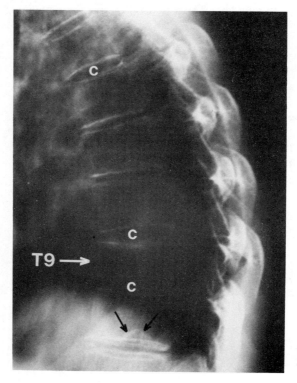

QUESTIONS:

1. What does the chest X-ray demonstrate?

2. What diagnoses should you consider?

3. What studies would you order?

4. What is the most likely diagnosis?

5. What risk factors are known to play a role in this problem?

6. What factors can we correct?

7. How would you manage this patient?

200 CASE STUDIES IN ENDOCRINOLOGY

ANSWERS:

1. The decreased bone mineral content gives a "washout" appearance (osteopenia) to the vertebral bodies. There is anterior wedging of T9, suggesting a compression fraction of the body of this vertebra. Ballooning of nuclei pulposi into weakened trabecular bone leads to concave deformities ("codfishing") of the vertebra (marked *C* on the X-ray). Localized herniation of the pulposus leads to Schmorl's node (the *arrows* point to this defect in T10).

2. Osteopenia on roentgenographs means at least a 30% decrease in trabecular bone mass. Most osteopenia relates to excessive loss of calcium from the bone. Causes include <u>hyperparathyroidism</u> (both primary and secondary), <u>primary osteoporosis</u> (postmenopausal, senile, involutional, idiopathic), and <u>secondary osteoporosis</u> (Cushing's syndrome, hyperthyroidism, alcoholism, multiple myeloma, immobilization, weightlessness, heparin-induced). Decreased mineralization from osteomalacia (rickets) also causes osteopenia.

3. <u>Order baseline serum chemistries that include calcium, phosphorus, albumin, alkaline phosphatase, BUN, creatinine, and electrolytes.</u> *[Serum Ca was 9.3 mg/dl; P, 3.9 mg/dl; albumin, 4.0 mg/dl; AP, 58 U (normal); BUN, 15; creatinine, 0.9 mg/dl; electrolytes, normal.]* <u>Order CBC</u>. Is there an underlying anemia to suggest myeloma? *[CBC normal.]*

4. <u>Primary (postmenopausal) osteoporosis</u> is the mostly likely diagnosis. Osteoporosis is the most common metabolic bone disease. It is an important cause of morbidity and mortality for the elderly. Osteoporotic bone has decreased bone volume (less mineralized matrix per unit volume) and less trabecular bridging, leading to fewer struts for support. The bone matrix appears to mineralize normally. Osteoporosis

SUDDEN-ONSET BACK PAIN 201

affects all bone, but trabecular bone (e.g., vertebrae, femoral head, distal radius) is much more involved than compact or cortical bone (e.g., shafts of long bones). The reduction in trabecular bone mass means that these affected bones are subject to collapse and fracture. The osteoporotic patient usually presents with compression fractures of vertebral bodies or fractures of distal radius or proximal femur.

5. The pathogenesis of osteoporosis is multifactorial. Bone mineral content reaches its maximum during the third decade of life. The amount of mineral deposited is dependent on body size (thin, petite-framed individuals have less mineral than large-framed individuals), sex (females have less than males), and race (Caucasians have less than Negroes). After the third decade there is a gradual reduction in body mineral content that is accelerated in the menopausal female. Estrogen has a vital role in preservation of mineral mass. Estrogen inhibits parathyroid hormone (PTH) effect on bone absorption. Estrogen deficiency is also associated with lower serum levels of 1,25-dihydroxyvitamin D, which leads to less intestinal absorption of calcium. These factors, plus an inadequate dietary intake of calcium by most adult women and possibly less sunlight exposure, are thought to be the reasons for the acceleration of mineral loss from the bone.

RISK FACTORS IN WOMEN FOR PRIMARY OSTEOPOROSIS

White or oriental race
Petite frame
Inadequate dietary intake of calcium
Early menopause or oophorectomy
Positive family history for osteoporosis
Alcohol abuse
Cigarette smoking
Sedentary life style

---

202 CASE STUDIES IN ENDOCRINOLOGY

Some patients have a significant family history of osteoporosis. Furthermore, chronic alcohol abuse and cigarette smoking compound these factors. Bone biopsy of osteoporotic patients confirms a multifactorial causation since some patients have increased bone resorption as well as decreased bone formation.

6. The risk factors that we can modify include: **a**) the dietary deficiency of calcium (add supplemental calcium); **b**) sedentary life style (begin a regular exercise program such as walking, biking, or jogging); **c**) early menopause or oophorectomy (prescribe estrogen); and **d**) alcohol and cigarette abuse (cut them out).

7. By the time we saw this patient, her pain had nearly resolved. However, treatment of newly diagnosed vertebral and symptomatic fractures requires bedrest, analgesics for pain, and local heat for relief of paravertebral muscle spasm. The muscle component often develops as the major component of chronic back pain. Avoid using narcotics for analgesia if possible. Early ambulation is recommended. If pain persists, back support in the form of a back brace is used. Patients are cautioned not to lift heavy objects and to bend at the knees instead of the waist when lifting objects. Exercise is strongly encouraged.

Unfortunately, there are no drugs which can provoke or increase the amount of normal bone mass. At present, all medications are given to retard the progression of the loss of mineral mass that accompanies aging. These medications include calcium and estrogen supplementation.

Elemental calcium (1.0-2.0 gm/day) taken as calcium carbonate is the safest, most economical, and convenient form of calcium supplementation. *[Generic $CaCO_3$ equivalent to 500 mg of Ca taken with each meal was prescribed for this* *patient.]* Drinking a quart of skim milk provides 1200 mg of calcium, but it is an option most women avoid. Oral calcium ingestion will correct any negative calcium balance and inhibit bone loss via resorption. It is as effective as any therapy in reducing height loss in patients who have crushed vertebra.

<u>Estrogen</u> is effective in treating osteoporosis. It retards bone loss by inhibiting PTH-induced resorption and by increasing gut absorption of calcium. Estrogen therapy has been demonstrated to reduce the fracture rate in osteoporosis, to reduce the loss of statural height, and to retard mineral loss from vertebral bodies as assessed by CT. At least 0.625 mg of conjugated estrogens is necessary to be effective. However, estrogens do have troublesome side effects including vaginal bleeding, increased risk of endometrial carcinoma, and tendency to fluid retention. Using a progestin (e.g., medroxyprogesterone acetate 10 mg each day for 5-10 days every third month on days 20-30) will produce withdrawal uterine bleeding and may decrease the risk of uterine cancer. Annual pelvic and breast exams are necessary, and all abnormal vaginal bleeding needs to be promptly investigated. The ideal candidate for estrogen therapy is the woman who has had a hysterectomy.

Synthetic salmon <u>calcitonin</u> may be used for the treatment of osteoporosis, but its cost (must be taken for months) and its route of administration (subcutaneous or intramuscular) make calcitonin less appealing for most patients. Sodium fluoride has also been used in treating osteoporosis. Fluoride increases bone mass but the bone is not normal. The doses used, 40-60 mg/day, are doses which also cause osteomalacia and secondary hyperparathyroidism. Fluoride therapy is still experimental and is not approved by the FDA for use in the treatment of osteoporosis.

204 CASE STUDIES IN ENDOCRINOLOGY

PEARLS:

1. The clinical presentation of osteoporosis relates to <u>pain and deformity associated with fracture</u>. Back pain is usually the symptom which brings the patient to the physician. The onset of pain may be sudden, aggravated by movement and weight bearing, and relieved by rest. Thoracic and lumbar vertebra are most affected (especially T12 and L1). The loss of vertebral height and anterior wedging leads to abnormal curvature colloquially known as "dowager's hump." Falls often cause femoral neck fractures or Colles' fracture of the wrist (both areas of considerable trabecular bone).

2. Laboratory findings are usually <u>not</u> specific for osteoporosis. <u>The serum Ca, P, and alkaline phosphatase are ususally normal</u>.

3. The patient who has the greatest risk for developing clinical osteoporosis (that is, fractures related to reduced bone mass) is the white, postmenopausal female who has a petite frame or had a petite frame at age 20 and now is obese.

4. Although postmenopausal or senile osteoporosis is the most common and least understood category of osteoporosis, there are several endocrine abnormalities associated with osteoporosis. These include estrogen deficiency during the premenopausal years, as in ovarian dysgenesis (Turner's syndrome) or premature menopause (surgical or idiopathic); testosterone deficiency; Cushing's syndrome; hyperthyroidism; and primary hyperparathyroidism.

5. All patients with osteoporosis are treated with oral calcium 1.0-2.0 gm/day. If there are no contraindications and the patient is perimenopausal, oral estrogen (taken cyclically as conjugated estrogen 0.625 mg on days 1-25 with oral progestin added at least every 3 months) is prescribed. For the patients who have had a hysterectomy, estrogen is taken

SUDDEN-ONSET BACK PAIN 205

daily. Exercise is encouraged and immobilization is only for the acute situation. If the response to therapy is poor, reconsider the diagnosis.

6. Vitamin D alone does not reduce height loss in patients with osteoporosis. However, pharmacological doses of vitamin D are used for patients with impaired bowel absorption of calcium. Generally these patients will have < 50 mg of urine calcium/24 hours (normal, 200-300 mg/day). These patients may well have osteomalacia in addition to osteoporosis on bone biopsy.

PITFALLS:

1. If there is no generalized osteopenia or if there are serum calcium abnormalities in a woman who presents with a compression vertebral fracture, one should consider the possibility of a <u>pathological fracture due to metastatic disease</u>. If there are anemia and vertebral fractures, myeloma should be excluded.

2. It is difficult to evaluate whether a treatment regimen is suitable or is working in an individual patient since our methods of quantitating bone mass are not very precise. Most recommended treatments are derived from epidemiological studies of populations of patients treated with different regimens. Photon absorption of the radius does not tell anything about the axial skeleton where the loss of mineral is the greatest. Computerized tomography of the vertebral body has the potential to be useful in following the treatment of osteoporosis.

3. Patients treated with calcium supplementation/estrogen replacement for osteoporosis should be followed yearly with

206 CASE STUDIES IN ENDOCRINOLOGY

serum calcium (hyperparathyroidism may show up) and with 24-hour urine calciums (vigorous treatment may lead to hypercalciuria; urine calciums ought not be > 250 mg/24 hours).

4. Vitamin D is not used alone for therapy of primary osteoporosis and is only occasionally used with oral calcium. Providing most patients with small doses of vitamin D2 (400 U/day) is sufficient to meet the requirements of vitamin D. High doses of vitamin D2 (e.g., ergocalciferol 50,000 U twice a week) can lead to hypercalciuria and possibly to hypercalcemia.

REFERENCES

Avioli LV: Osteoporosis: pathogenesis and therapy. In Avioli LV, Krane SM (eds): Metabolic Bone Disease. New York, Academic Press, 1977, pp 307-385.

Lindsay R. Osteoporosis. In Krieger DT, Bardin CW (eds): Current Therapy in Endocrinology 1985-1986. Toronto, B.C. Decker, 1985, pp 322-324.

Raisz LG: Osteoporosis. J Am Geriatr Soc 30:127, 1982.

Singer FR: Metabolic bone disease. In Felig P, Baxter JD, Broadus AE, Frohman LA (eds): Endocrinology and Metabolism. New York, McGraw-Hill, 1981, pp 1081-1118.

FACIAL SWELLING AND DIABETES MELLITUS

CASE 26: L.W., a 17-year-old high school student, presented because of swelling and pain over the left side of his face. For the last 2 weeks, he had experienced increased thirst, frequent urination, and generalized weakness. He had noticed that the left side of his face appeared fuller over the last 24 hours. Because of nausea and facial and abdominal pain, he came to the emergency room. His past medical history was unremarkable. His usual weight was 160 lb. There was no family history of diabetes, thyroid, or other metabolic disease.

On exam, this young black man was tachypneic (rate, 26/min); weight, 151 lb; height, 69 inches; pulse 110/min; BP, 90/60 (lying), 70/50 (standing); temperature, 100.8°F. He was acutely ill and asking for water, but oriented as to time, place, and person. His skin was dry and had decreased turgor. His breath was fruity. Tissue around the left eye was edematous. Tenderness was noted to deep palpation over the left malar area inferior to the orbit. No lesions could be seen in the nose, nor was any discharge noted. The left eye moved normally, but the patient noted diplopia when he used both eyes. No oral lesions were noted. Chest, abdomen, rectal, and neurological exams were normal.

208   CASE STUDIES IN ENDOCRINOLOGY

ENDOCRINE CLUE: Urinalysis: 4+ glucose; 3+ ketones; specific gravity, 1.015; pH, 5.0; negative for protein and hemoglobin; no cells seen. Serum electrolytes: Na, 130 mEq/l; K, 5.5 mEq/l; HCO_3, 13 mEq/l; Cl, 110 mEq/l; BUN, 37 mg/dl; ketones, positive at 1:8 dilution; plasma glucose, 353 mg/dl. Arterial blood gases: pH, 7.20; PO_2, 98; and PCO_2, 30.

QUESTIONS:

1. What is this patient's diagnosis?

2. What factors must you consider that might have precipitated this man's illness?

3. What other studies should you order?

4. How would you manage this patient?

5. Twelve hours later, he cannot move his left eye. What would you do?

6. After noting the results of the studies (response to Question #5), what caused the ophthalmoplegia?

7. How would you treat this problem?

210   CASE STUDIES IN ENDOCRINOLOGY

ANSWERS:

1. Diabetic ketoacidosis (DKA) is obvious. Clinical symptoms of uncontrolled diabetic acidosis include excessive thirst and dry mouth, polyuria, weight loss, air-hunger, nausea (often with vomiting), weakness, muscle aches, headache, abdominal pain, and central nervous system depression with drowsiness and stupor which may progress to coma. There are often symptoms related to a coexistent infection. Signs of DKA include: dehydration with dry mucous membranes, dry skin with poor turgor, sunken eyeballs, tachypnea (often deep and labored), a characteristic fruity odor to the breath, tachycardia, and hypotension.

   The CLUE contains the laboratory findings of DKA: blood glucose is > 300 mg/dl; serum bicarbonate, < 15 mEq/l; arterial blood pH, < 7.30; plasma acetone, positive at 1:2 dilution or greater. The serum potassium may be low, normal, or high, but the total body potassium is depleted. The serum sodium is usually normal but may be low if the serum is lipemic.

2. Infection is the most likely precipitating cause. Fever and DKA mean infection until proven otherwise. In this case, the differential includes sinusitis, facial cellulitis, orbital cellulitis, or tooth abscess. Abdominal pain is common in DKA (may mimic acute abdomen), but the physical exam in this patient did not point to an abdominal process. Although pneumonia and urinary tract infection should be considered in any patient with DKA, they seem unlikely in this patient.

3. Other studies needed include: CBC (infection, underlying hematologic disorder); serum for creatinine (possible prerenal azotemia with elevated BUN); calcium (may be low in pancreatitis); phosphorus (low P often causes severe weakness); magnesium; blood and urine cultures (infection);

FACIAL SWELLING AND DIABETES MELLITUS 211

and E C G (baseline). X-rays of sinuses and orbits are particularly important in this patient.

4. A quick response is most important, and you should not wait for every lab result before instituting therapy. The management of DKA requires fluid replacement, insulin administration, correction of electrolyte abnormalities, and investigation of precipitating causes. If possible, the patient should be treated in an acute care unit where close monitoring is available. Since much of the therapy listed below is administered concomitantly and multiple blood determinations are needed to optimize patient care, a well-planned flow sheet is a necessity.

Fluid replacement: An intravenous line using at least a 19-gauge needle or catheter is established. The typical adult DKA patient needs 6-10 liters to replete his or her fluid status. Normal saline is administrated to the hypotensive patient, whereas most patients are given 0.45% saline solution (1/2 normal saline) since the plasma osmolality is already elevated (but not as high as in hyperosmolar coma). The infusion rate should be rapid (1000 ml for the first 30 minutes; 1000 ml for next hour; then, 300-500 ml/hour over the first 24 hours). The rate varies depending on urine output, blood pressure, and the circulatory response to a large volume load. As soon as the blood sugar falls below 250 mg/dl, then dextrose 5% (D5/W) is infused.

Insulin administration: There are many regimens for giving regular insulin. Each works as long as there is intensive hourly monitoring of the patient's status and recognition of how prior treatment has worked. The use of bolus intravenous insulin, subcutaneous insulin every 2 hours, hourly intramuscular insulin, or continuous intravenous drip (with or without a starting bolus) does not matter; paying close attention to the patient does. Because hypokalemia and

212 CASE STUDIES IN ENDOCRINOLOGY

hypoglycemia are less frequent with "low dose" regimens, the author prefers to give 10 U of regular insulin (intravenous push) followed by a constant infusion of 6 U/hour (up to 12 U/hour if there is infection, etc.). If there is no response in the blood sugar (expect a 5-10% fall in plasma glucose each hour) or if the acidemia is not being corrected within 3 or 4 hours, then higher insulin doses are used.

Regular insulin is not stopped when the plasma glucose falls below 250 mg/dl, but dextrose 5% is started and the amount of insulin infused per hour may be decreased (but continued until the acidosis is corrected). Intermediate insulin should not be given until the patient is stabilized and able to drink and eat food.

Correct electrolyte abnormalities: Because of the acidemia and osmotic diuresis of DKA, a typical patient has lost 600 mEq of sodium, 400 mEq of potassium, 400 mEq of chloride, 400 mEq of bicarbonate, and 100 mEq of phosphate. If the initial serum K is > 5.5 mEq/l, then no KCl is added to the initial iv fluids. If the serum K is normal, then sufficient KCl is added to each liter of fluid so that no more than 40 mEq/hour is infused. If the serum K is < 3.5 mEq/l, then 40-80 mEq/hour is given with close monitoring of ECG and serum K determinations at least every 2 hours. Both the serum K and serum phosphorus fall after fluid and insulin are started, and a portion of potassium replacement may be given as potassium phosphate. Any suggestion of renal impairment means less aggressive K and phosphate replacement.

Investigate the precipitating cause: This is necessary since any overt or occult infection can lead to DKA. *[In this patient, the roentgenograms showed clouding of the right maxillary sinus and indistinct medial aspect of the orbital rim at the ethmoid sinus suggesting bone erosion.]* The diagnosis of

FACIAL SWELLING AND DIABETES MELLITUS   213

sinusitis, probably of bacterial origin, was made and the patient was started on penicillin and gentamycin.

4. The possibility of diabetic third nerve palsy seems unlikely in the presence of a localized process. Most likely, this represents an extension of the infectious process to the orbital apex or possible invasion of the cavernous sinus and/or thrombosis of the cavernous sinus. <u>You examine the patient thoroughly</u>. A dark, necrotic middle nasal turbinate is found. <u>You scrape the lesion and examine the specimen</u>. The following photomicrograph depicts the findings.

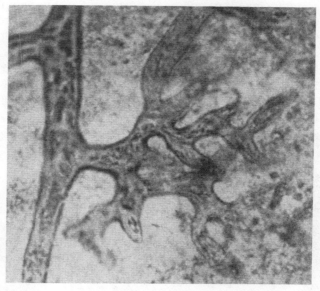

5. <u>Mucormycosis (rhinocerebral)</u>. The phycomycetes cause a rare and often fatal fungal disease that almost always occurs in the compromised host (diabetic ketoacidosis is by far the most common condition). The fungus (<u>Rhizopus</u>, <u>Mucor</u>, and <u>Asidia</u>) gains access by inhalation, infects nasal mucosa, and spreads by direct extension to palate, sinuses, and orbit. The

predilection of the organism to invade blood-vessel walls causes thrombosis and tissue infarction leading to the clinical picture of dark, necrotic lesions (black eschar) of the palate and nasal turbinates that rarely bleed. The fungus appears in the tissues as nonseptate hyphae that are irregular and tend to branch at right angles (see photomicrograph).

6. The key points in treatment of mucormycosis include: a) <u>early diagnosis</u> (direct microscopic exam of material mixed with 2-3 drops of 10-20% KOH looking for large, branching, nonseptate hyphae); b) <u>systemic antifungal therapy</u> (<u>start amphotericin B</u>); c) <u>aggressive surgical debridement</u> (consult the ENT surgeon and ophthalmologist). Excision of devitalized tissue is essential (the fungus thrives in necrotic tissue); d) <u>treatment of any concurrent bacterial infection since the necrotic tissue is often infected with bacteria</u> (culture for bacteria as well as fungus); and e) <u>control of underlying disease</u>. This patient survived but not without cost (see photograph below).

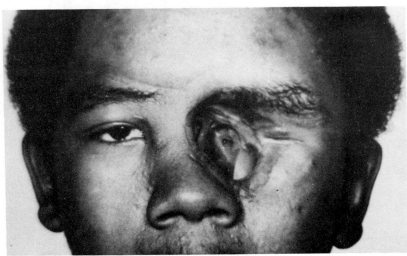

FACIAL SWELLING AND DIABETES MELLITUS 215

PEARLS:

1. DKA is the most common endocrine emergency. Immediate diagnosis and aggressive management with careful attention to detail can reduce the mortality of this life-threatening disorder to below 2%.

2. Certain risk factors that predispose patients with DKA to higher mortality include: <u>delay in making the diagnosis or instituting appropriate therapy</u>, <u>advanced age</u>, <u>deep coma</u>, <u>uremia</u>, and <u>myocardial infarction</u>.

3. The serum phosphorus may fall below 1.0 mg/dl during therapy. Patients with hypophosphatemia on admission are at risk to develop severe hypophosphatemia with insulin therapy and are most likely to benefit from P supplementation. Phosphate may be given at the rate of 10-15 mmol/hour in the form of a buffered potassium phosphate solution (3 mmol P/ml and 4 mEq K/ml), adding 5 ml of this solution to each liter of intravenous fluid.

4. Ptosis, third cranial nerve palsy, and sparing of the pupil suggest diabetic mononeuropathy (this requires no treatment and has a excellent chance to resolve spontaneously over a few months). Losing the pupillary response or anisocoria points to a more ominous process (e.g., mass lesion, aneurysm, subarachnoid hemorrhage).

5. Transferrin (with measurable iron-binding capacity) plays a critical role in preventing fungal growth in serum. The acidosis that occurs during DKA leads to decreased iron-binding capacity and thus abolishes the fungal growth inhibitory activity of serum.

216   CASE STUDIES IN ENDOCRINOLOGY

PITFALLS:

1. The nitroprusside reaction (crushed Acetest® tablet on which one drop of diluted plasma is reacted for 2 minutes) detects acetone and acetoacetate but not ß-hydroxybutyrate, the major ketone body in DKA. Undiluted serum may give a strong acetone reaction in states of starvation alone. Serum is considered positive at a 1:2 dilution.

2. The use of bicarbonate therapy in DKA is controversial. There are some good reasons to avoid bicarbonate administration. With acute alkalinization, there is a paradoxical fall of cerebral spinal fluid pH, leading to CNS depression (worsening of stupor/coma) and a shift in the hemoglobin oxygen disassociation curve (Bohr effect) leading to tissue hypoxia. However, if the pH is < 7.1 and death is near, then 2 ampules of sodium bicarbonate (144 mEq of Na and HCO_3) should be added to a liter of hypotonic saline 0.45% and infused over 1 hour. Do not give bolus bicarbonate. The goal is to raise the pH to 7.20-7.25. Lactate is not used in DKA since some patients, particularly hypotensive subjects, already have elevated blood lactate levels.

3. If phosphorus is used in treating DKA, you should measure serum calcium every 4-6 hours since hyperphosphatemia will cause hypocalcemia and possible tetany. Addition of PO_4 is contraindicated in renal insufficiency.

4. Remember that serum creatinine levels as measured by colorimetric determination are increased in DKA. An accurate assessment of creatinine status must come from other methodologies (e.g., enzymatic techniques).

5. Failure to treat bacterial infections that are superimposed upon phycomycotic lesions leads to increased morbidity and mortality.

REFERENCES

Artis WM, Fountain JA, Delcher HK, et al: A mechanism of susceptibility to mucormycosis in diabetic ketoacidosis: transferrin and iron availability. Diabetes 31:1109, 1982.

Ferry AP, Abedi S: Diagnosis and management of rhino-orbitocerebral mucormycosis (phycomycosis). Ophthalmology 90:1096, 1983.

Fisher JN, Shahshahani MN, Kitabchi AE: Diabetic ketoacidosis: low dose insulin therapy by various routes. N Engl J Med 297:238, 1977.

Foster DW, McGarry JD: The metabolic derangements and treatment of diabetic ketoacidosis. N Engl J Med 309:159, 1983.

Kilpatrick CJ, Speer AG, Tress BM, et al: Rhinocerebral mucormycosis. Med J Aust 1:308, 1983.

Lehrer RI, Howard DH, Sypherd PS, et al: Mucormycosis. Ann Intern Med 93:93, 1980.

Pillsbury HC, Fischer ND: Rhinocerebral mucormycosis. Arch Otolaryngol 103:600, 1977.

Ranguel-Guerra R, Martinez HR, Saenz C: Mucomycosis: report of 11 cases. Arch Neurol 42:578, 1985.

Schade DS, Eaton RP, Alberti KGMM, Johnston DG: Diabetic Coma: Ketoacidotic and Hyperosmolar. Albuquerque, University of New Mexico Press, 1981.

DIABETES MELLITUS TYPE II

CASE 27: B.P., a 41-year-old housewife, recently experienced a 2-week history of increased thirst, frequent urination, and a 4-lb weight loss. Because her older brother had diabetes mellitus, she checked her urine using Testape® and found the strip to be dark green. She had been in good health. She denied fever, dysuria, back pain, cough, myalgias, or headache. Her menses were regular. She had delivered three term infants weighing over 8 lb (none over 9.1 lb). The family history was positive for diabetes mellitus (a brother taking an oral hypoglycemic agent and mother with "borderline" diabetes). There were no other known endocrine disorders.

The patient weighed 145 lb; her height was 62 inches; BP, 130/85; pulse, 75/min and regular. Other than mild obesity, the examination was normal.

ENDOCRINE CLUE: Classifying the diabetes helps you focus on the best approach to manage the patient.

Diabetes Mellitus (DM)	Type I	Type II
Age of onset (yr)	< 40 (often < 20)	> 40
Family history of DM	Rare	Common (95%)
Ketosis prone	Yes	No
Specific HLA associations	Yes	No
Obesity	Rare	Common (80%)
Insulin sensitivity	Sensitive	Resistant
Requires insulin	Yes	Generally not

DIABETES MELLITUS TYPE II   219

QUESTIONS:

1. What are the criteria for the diagnosis of diabetes mellitus?

2. What studies would you order on this patient?

3. After reviewing the results of these studies, how would you manage her problem?

4. How many calories should you prescribe for her each day?

5. After 2 months of treatment, she is no longer symptomatic but continues to have fasting blood glucoses of 150 mg/dl or greater. What would you recommend?

220   CASE STUDIES IN ENDOCRINOLOGY

ANSWERS:

1. Diabetes mellitus is easily diagnosed when there is unequivocal elevation of the plasma glucose (> 200 mg/dl) with classical symptoms of polyuria, polydipsia, polyphagia, and weight loss. This patient meets these criteria. Some patients may not have this degree of hyperglycemia or these symptoms. In these patients an oral glucose tolerance test (GTT) is used to establish the diagnosis of diabetes mellitus. The National Diabetes Study Group has made recommendations for the standardization of testing and has established criteria for the diagnosis of diabetes mellitus which are very useful. By these criteria, diabetes mellitus is present when:
   a) Fasting plasma glucose is > 140 mg/dl on two occasions or
   b) Fasting plasma glucose is < 140 mg/dl and 2-hour plasma glucose > 200 mg/dl with one intervening value is > 200 mg/dl following a 75-gm glucose load (GTT).

2. You order routine laboratory studies that include serum for glucose, BUN, creatinine, electrolytes, fasting triglycerides, and cholesterol, and urine for urinalysis. *[Abnormal results were plasma glucose, 280 mg/dl; triglycerides, 300 mg/dl; cholesterol, 250 mg/dl; urine glucose, 5% with no ketones.]* You may order a glycosylated hemoglobin (Hgb A1c) as a baseline measurement to follow diabetic control in the future.

3. The patient has type II diabetes mellitus. The family history is positive for diabetes; she has hyperglycemia and glycosuria without ketosis; she is middle aged and overweight. Management of her problem begins with diet, exercise, and weight reduction. Early in the stage of type II diabetes, the problem is mostly insulin resistance. Obesity itself causes insulin resistance (a common problem for > 80% of type II patients). This patient needs to learn the

DIABETES MELLITUS TYPE II 221

symptoms, signs, and possible complications of diabetes and to understand why you are putting her on a 1100-calorie diet, why weight reduction might cure her diabetes, and why diet is so critical to her health. <u>Exercise</u> aids weight reduction. Walking (4-5 miles/day), biking, or swimming should be encouraged. The team approach (physician, nurse clinician, nutritionist) helps considerably in management. <u>Self-monitoring of blood glucose</u> (home monitoring) and <u>glycosylated hemoglobin</u> (Hgb A1 or Hgb A1c) are two helpful tools that aid in managing the patient with diabetes.

4. <u>The number of calories (kcal) recommended is based on body weight and activity.</u> Ideal body weight (IBW) for adult females with a medium frame approximates 100 lb plus 5 lb for each inch over 5 feet. Thus, this patient's IBW is 110 lb. For a small frame, deduct 10% from the IBW; for a large frame, add 10% of the IBW. For medium-frame males, the IBW is 106 lb plus 6 lb for each inch over 5 feet. Deduct or add 10% of the IBW for a small or large frame, respectively.

The total calorie requirement each day is the <u>sum of the basal requirements plus the activity requirements</u>. Basal calorie requirement is figured as the IBW times a factor of 10 (IBW x 10). The calorie requirement based on activity for a sedentary life style is the IBW x 3; for moderate activity, IBW x 5; and for heavy work, IBW x 10. <u>A total of 1650 calories is needed to maintain this patient's weight.</u> [1000 calories (basal requirement) plus 550 calories (activity requirement assuming moderate activity).]

Since she needs to reduce her weight, decreasing her total calorie intake to 500 calories/day less than the maintenance requirement will produce a 1-lb weight loss each week (minus 1000 calories/day will give a 2-lb weight reduction each week). <u>Prescribe a 1100-calorie diet.</u> A well-balanced diet eaten regularly at breakfast, lunch, and dinner (bedtime

222 CASE STUDIES IN ENDOCRINOLOGY

snack for those patients receiving insulin) is necessary. A diet composed of 50% carbohydrate, 20% protein, and 30% fat is reasonable, but food preferences and socio-economic situations should be used to determine the precise regimen. Consultation with the dietician is quite helpful.

5. Even though she is asymptomatic, the fasting blood sugar (FBS) is high. What to do next depends on whether the patient is following her diet and losing weight. If her weight is 140 lb, then stress the importance of adherence to the diet and weight reduction. If she has lost weight to 120 lb and still has an elevated FBS and increased glycosylated hemoglobin, then addition of an oral hypoglycemic agent should be considered. There are a variety of sulfonylureas from which to choose. Some of the frequently prescribed agents include:

Agent	Daily Dose (mg)	Cost/Day @ Maximum Dose
Tolazamide (generic)	250-1000	$0.75
Chlopropamide	100-500	$0.65
Glyburide	2.5-20	$1.25
Glipizide	5-40	$1.30

If diet, weight reduction, and oral agents fail to control diabetes, then insulin administration may be necessary.

PEARLS:

1. Most type II diabetic patients do not need supplemental insulin. Prescribing insulin leads to a vicious circle in which insulin lowers blood glucose, stimulates appetite, and promotes weight gain, leading to more insulin resistance and finally a return to hyperglycemia.

DIABETES MELLITUS TYPE II   223

2. Several years after the onset of type II diabetes, some patients lose the ability to secrete insulin and become insulin dependent as well as insulin resistant. These patients require insulin. Another indication for insulin treatment in type II diabetes is to cover acute stress situations such as surgery, infection, myocardial infarction, etc.

3. Sulfonylurea drugs may be used to treat the hyperglycemia in type II diabetes, but again <u>use of these agents in the noncompliant obese subject is usually doomed to fail</u>. Up to 60% of the patients have an initial good response of blood glucose, but sulfonylureas produce effective long-term results in only 20-30% of patients.

4. Factors that favor success with sulfonylurea therapy in type II diabetes include <u>onset of diabetes after age 40</u>, <u>normal body weight or obese</u>, <u>known duration of diabetes < 5 years</u>, and <u>no prior history of insulin therapy or well controlled on < 40 U of insulin/day</u>. Patients who are underweight are likely to be insulin dependent and usually have a high primary failure rate to sulfonylureas.

5. Women with type II diabetes often give a history of large infants (> 8 lb). Gestational diabetes may or may not have been recognized.

6. A small subset of type II patients (<u>maturity-onset diabetes of youth or MODY</u>) differ from classic type II diabetics. MODY patients develop diabetes at an early age, have a family history of diabetes (autosomal dominant), and respond well to sulfonylurea therapy.

224   CASE STUDIES IN ENDOCRINOLOGY

PITFALLS:

1. Glucose tolerance testing is <u>not</u> recommended in the following circumstances: **a**) <u>when fasting hyperglycemia is already present</u>, **b**) <u>in hospitalized patients, acutely ill patients, or patients who are physically inactive</u> (e.g., bedridden), or **c**) <u>subjects taking medications such as diuretics, propranolol, dilantin, glucocorticoids, estrogens, and birth control pills</u>.

2. The GTT should be performed only on subjects who have been on an unrestricted diet containing at least 300 gm of carbohydrate/day and who have been physically active for 3 days prior to the test. A 75-gm glucose load should be administrated in the morning after a 10-hour fast.   The patient should remained seated and should not smoke during the study. Blood is obtained at 0, 30, 60, 90, and 120 minutes.

3. Some patients have impaired glucose tolerance (fasting plasma glucose < 140 mg/dl; 2-hour plasma glucose > 140 mg/dl but < 200 mg/dl; and an intervening value > 200 mg/dl) following the 75-gm load.   These subjects have an abnormality in glucose metabolism intermediate between normal and overt diabetes.   It may worsen to diabetes, improve toward normal, or remain unchanged on serial testing. <u>It is best to label these patients as having impaired glucose tolerance and not diabetes mellitus</u>.

4. Chlorpropamide's prolonged duration of action (24-60 hours) increases the risk of hypoglycemia.   Chlorpropamide also may augment the release of vasopressin (ADH), leading to hyponatremia and possible water intoxication.

5. Up to 50% of patients with type II diabetes initially controlled with sulfonylureas can be taken off these agents

DIABETES MELLITUS TYPE II   225

and still maintain control of the diabetes (provided they adhere to a diet).

REFERENCES

Fajans SS: The adult diabetic patient. In Krieger DT, Bardin CW (eds): Current Therapy in Endocrinology 1985-1986. Toronto, B.C. Decker, 1985, pp 245-254.

Koenig RJ, Peterson CM, Jones RL, et al: Correlation of glucose regulation and hemoglobin A1c in diabetes mellitus. N Engl J Med 295:417, 1976.

Lebovitz HE, Feinglos MN: Sulfonylurea drugs: mechanism of antidiabetic action and therapeutic usefulness. Diabetes Care 1:189, 1978.

Lebovitz HE: Clinical utility of oral hypoglycemic agents in the management of patients with noninsulin-dependent diabetes mellitus. Am J Med 75 (Suppl 5B):94, 1983.

National Diabetes Data Group: Classification and diagnosis of diabetes mellitus and other categories of glucose intolerance. Diabetes 28:1039, 1979.

Sonksen PH, Judd SL, Lowy C: Home monitoring of blood glucose. Method for improving diabetic control. Lancet 1:729, 1979.

DIABETES AND CONTROL

CASE 28: S.S., a 24-year-old single woman, presents for regulation and management of diabetes. At the age of 16 years, she developed diabetes mellitus. She had adhered to a 2000-calorie diabetic diet, had taken a single dose of NPH insulin (gradually increased from 24 to 48 U each AM), and had checked her urine with reagent strips each morning (usually 1+ to 3+). Because she had no obvious problems related to diabetes and had moved from another city, she had not seen a physician in 2 years. She denied any insulin reactions, polyuria, weight change, diarrhea, paresthesias, or visual difficulty. There was no family history of diabetes mellitus.

On examination, she weighed 125 lb; height, 64 inches; BP, 125/80; pulse, 70 and regular. The examination revealed sparsely scattered dot hemorrhages in both retinas, absent ankle deep tendon reflexes, decreased vibratory sensation over the feet, and several nontender lesions over the lower legs (see CLUE).

ENDOCRINE CLUE:

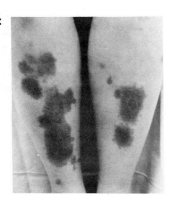

DIABETES AND CONTROL   227

QUESTIONS:

1. What does the photograph demonstrate?

2. What complications of diabetes mellitus does she manifest?

3. What is glycosylated hemoglobin and how it is used in patients with diabetes?

4. What are the goals of managing a patient with diabetes?

5. What is good diabetic control?

6. How would you manage this patient?

228 CASE STUDIES IN ENDOCRINOLOGY

ANSWERS:

1. Necrobiosis lipoidica diabeticorum (NLD). NLD is a chronic, asymptomatic lesion most often seen in females which typically involves the anterior surface of the lower extremities. The areas are generally flat, large (> 1 cm), and yellow-brown with well-circumscribed borders. Early lesions are slightly raised and have a dusky red appearance. Pathologic changes in the lower dermis lead to loss of normal structure (necrobiosis) with late changes of giant inflammatory cells such as histiocytes and foam cells (lipoidica). The precise correlation with diabetes and the pathogenesis of the lesion remain controversial. There is no satisfactory therapy.

2. Complications are diabetic skin disease (necrobiosis lipoidica diabeticorum), diabetic retinopathy (the blot or dot hemorrhages without new vessel formation indicate nonproliferative retinopathy), and diabetic neuropathy (loss of deep tendon reflexes and vibratory sensation to lower extremities signal a sensory polyneuropathy). Whether she has nephropathy is unknown.

3. Nonenzymatic addition of glucose to proteins occurs in the body and in the test tube. High glucose concentrations favor the formation of these stable glycoproteins. When the hemoglobin A is glycosylated, Hgb A1c is formed. Normally, Hgb A1c represents less than than 6% of the total hemoglobin (the range varies with different assay techniques). Technically, it is easier to measure glycosylated hemoglobin as Hgb A1 (normal values are < 8%), so Hgb A1 is more often assayed than is Hgb A1c. In poorly controlled diabetics, Hgb A1 accounts for > 12% of the total hemoglobin. Glycosylated hemoglobin correlates with the degree of glycemia during the last 6-8 weeks (the half-life of erythrocytes is about 120 days) and gives an integrated value (in contrast to blood

DIABETES AND CONTROL 229

sugar which fluctuates widely). When properly performed, the glycosylated hemoglobin is helpful in confirming whether the control of blood sugar has been "on the average" what the patient says it has been. Whether glycosylation of proteins in general has any direct role in the pathogenesis of diabetic complications (micro- or macrovascular disease) is uncertain.

4. The ideal management of diabetes would lead to a <u>normal life style</u>; <u>normal glucose, fat, and protein metabolism</u>; <u>avoidance of hypoglycemia</u>; <u>prevention of long-term complications</u>; and <u>satisfactory psychosocial adaptation to living with a chronic disease</u>. These goals can be achieved in acute diabetes (diabetic ketoacidosis, hyperosmolar coma), but are usually only transiently achieved in the day-to-day care of patients with diabetes mellitus. Sixty years of experience with insulin therapy have not prevented the long-term complications of this disorder. There are abundant laboratory data to suggest that achievement of euglycemia is the best way to prevent these complications. Although 20% of patients with diabetes mellitus never develop complications, there is no way to detect these "protected" patients in advance. The author believes that the best method to avoid long-term complications of diabetes is to maintain the blood sugar as close to normal as possible. If the physician's attitude is lackadaisical, this philosophy is transferred to the patient and reflects how he or she will handle his or her diabetes.

5. <u>Control is difficult to define</u>. Ideal control mimics the plasma glucose variation in normal subjects. The level of hyperglycemia must be arbitrarily set for each patient and his or her particular circumstances. For example, the degree of hyperglycemia permitted may be greater for a 75-year-old subject than for an otherwise healthy 23-year-old individual mainly because of the risks of hypoglycemia (insulin reaction) in the elderly. Since we can quantitate

230 CASE STUDIES IN ENDOCRINOLOGY

biochemical parameters, they are most often used as indices of control. These biochemical criteria are useful in assessing diabetic control.

Descriptive	FBS	2-Hour Postcibal Blood Glucose	Hgb A1	Serum Cholesterol
Excellent (great)	65-115	< 140	< 8	< 200
Acceptable (good)	< 140	< 200	< 8	< 230
Fair (Not good)	< 200	< 230	< 10	< 250
Poor (bad)	> 200	> 230	> 10	> 250

In general, a preprandial blood glucose level of < 140 mg/dl represents acceptable control. <u>Strong motivation and good education make the difference between good and poor diabetic control.</u> Economics can also be a factor.

6. Before you can manage this patient effectively, you need more information about her urine and serum and some idea how well her diabetes is controlled. <u>Order urinalysis, plasma glucose, serum electrolytes, BUN, creatinine, fasting triglycerides, cholesterol, and hemoglobin A1 (glycosylated Hgb).</u> *[The urine showed 3+ glucose, no protein or ketones. A random blood sugar was 340 mg/dl; triglycerides, 300 mg/dl; cholesterol, 240 mg/dl; and glycosylated Hgb, 13% (normal for this assay, 4-8%).]* Thus, over the last 6 to 8 weeks her control was poor.

DIABETES AND CONTROL   231

Some guidelines are needed when treating the diabetic patient:

a) <u>The patient must be an active participant in the care of her diabetes</u>. She is responsible for adhering to diet, taking insulin injections, and for testing and recording her blood glucose or urine sugar before meals and bedtime.

b) <u>Monitoring these variables is the only way to assess whether the insulin regimen is controlling the diabetes</u>. Home monitoring of blood glucose (Dextrostix®, Chemstrip bG®, etc.) is especially helpful in planning therapy. Finger puncture with disposable lancets using an automatic, spring-loaded apparatus (Autolet®, Autoclick®, etc.) facilitates blood sampling and is practically painless. The reagent strips for checking the blood glucose are reliable when care is taken to follow directions, but they cost $40-$50 per 100 strips.

c) <u>Insulin treatment should be designed to give an adequate amount of insulin throughout the day and night</u>. In most patients with "brittle" or type I diabetes, one injection of an intermediate-acting insulin will not control the blood sugar throughout the day. Increasing the dose to > 60 U/day as a single injection greatly increases the risk of hypoglycemia. To avoid these problems, try splitting the insulin into two injections of intermediate insulin (before breakfast and before the evening meal) and add a short-acting insulin (regular, Semilente®, or Actrapid®). In theory, it is possible to "cover" the entire 24-hour day with such a "split-mixed" regimen.

232   CASE STUDIES IN ENDOCRINOLOGY

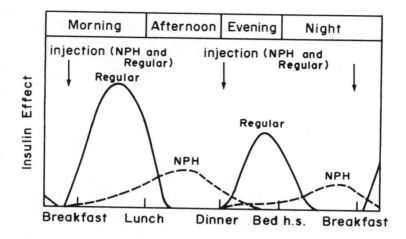

Split-Mixed Program of Twice a Day Insulin. Regular and intermediate insulin are taken together as a single injection 30-60 minutes prior to breakfast and to the evening meal.

Handouts containing recommendations for diabetic management and algorithms such as the one given on the following page are helpful in allowing patients to adjust their own split-mixed program and thereby to become responsible for their own diabetes care on a day-to-day basis. Try to normalize fasting blood sugar first. Whenever there is hypoglycemia (insulin reactions or blood glucose < 60 mg/dl), reduce the insulin dose.

DIABETES AND CONTROL   233

HYPERGLYCEMIA NOT EXPLAINED BY UNUSUAL DIET/EXERCISE/INSULIN

If the blood glucose before lunch is > 140 mg/dl for 3 days in a row, begin on day 4 to increase the morning regular insulin by _____ units.

If the blood glucose before the evening meal is > 140 mg/dl for 3 days in a row, begin on day 4 to increase the morning NPH (or Lente) insulin by _____ units.

If the blood glucose at bedtime is > 140 mg/dl for 3 days in a row, begin on day 4 to increase the evening regular insulin by _____ units.

If the blood glucose before breakfast is > 140 mg/dl for 3 days in a row, begin on day 4 to increase the evening NPH insulin by _____ units.

Small changes of 1-5 U of each insulin (usually 10% of the daily dose) are written in the blanks and a copy of the algorithm is given to the patient. For the patient who does not monitor his or her blood sugar, urine sugars are monitored and the statement would read: "If urine sugars are positive (record in percent) before . . ., then increase appropriate insulin by 5-10% for each percent spill . . . ."

PEARLS:

1. Probably nowhere else in medical therapeutics are there more ways to manage a problem than in diabetes mellitus.

2. The most crucial time to share the philosophy of management as well as the specifics on how to achieve desired goals is immediately after the diagnosis is made (first office visit, first hospitalization). It is very difficult to change life habits once they are established.

234   CASE STUDIES IN ENDOCRINOLOGY

3. Cutting the strips in half helps the cost of home monitoring but does not help for those who use a reflectometer (the entire width of the strip is needed to get accurate readings).

4. If the patient cannot afford blood glucose monitoring of his or her diabetes, then urine is checked before meals and at bedtime using either tablets (Clinitest® 2-drop method) or reagent strips (these are easier to use). A "double-void" specimen (empty bladder first, then urinate 15-30 minutes later and check this specimen) is particularly necessary in the morning. The goal for control using urine is aglycosuria with very infrequent insulin reactions.

5. A team approach which uses the expertise of a dietician, diabetic teaching nurse, and physician is ideal. A checklist helps to insure that the patient receives optimal instructions.

6. Abrupt increases in fasting levels of plasma glucose occuring between 5 and 9 AM without antecedent hypoglycemia is called <u>the dawn phenomenon</u>. The dawn phenomenon is common in insulin-dependent (type I) and non-insulin dependent (type II) diabetes mellitus.

PITFALLS:

1. A drawback of using glycosylated hemoglobin is that standards are not available to compare various assay techniques. Also, any process that increases the turnover of erythrocytes affects its interpretation.

2. Normal levels for glycosylated hemoglobin vary depending upon the assay; hemoglobin A1c values are lower than hemoglobin A1 values.

DIABETES AND CONTROL 235

3. The time to initiate regular diet, weight control, insulin dosage, etc., is not when the patient finally presents with symptomatic neuropathy, claudication, or loss of vision. Preventing these complications requires a committed approach early in the disease. <u>Patient education is a primary factor in achieving adequate control.</u>

4. Patients receiving insulin may develop rebound hyperglycemia following unrecognized hypoglycemia during their sleep. This set of events is called the <u>Somogyi phenomenon.</u> Reducing the insulin dose helps the morning hyperglycemia.

REFERENCES

Bolli GB, Gerich JE: The "dawn phenomenon"--a common occurrence in both non-insulin-dependent and insulin-dependent diabetes. <u>N Engl J Med</u> 310:746, 1984.

Fajans SS: The adult diabetic patient. In Krieger DT, Bardin CW (eds): <u>Current Therapy in Endocrinology 1985-1986.</u> Toronto, BC Decker, 1985, pp 245-254.

Felig P: The endocrine pancreas: diabetes mellitus. In Felig P, Baxter JD, Broadus AE, Frohman LA (eds): <u>Endocrinology and Metabolism.</u> New York, McGraw-Hill, 1981, pp 761-868.

Galloway JA, Bressler R: Insulin treatment in diabetes. <u>Med Clin North Am</u> 62:663, 1978.

Koenig RJ, Peterson CM, Jones RL, et al: Correlation of glucose regulation and hemoglobin A1c in diabetes mellitus. <u>N Engl J Med</u> 295:417, 1976.

Skyler JS, Skyler DL, Seigler DE, et al: Algorithms for the adjustment of insulin dosage by patients who moniter blood glucose. <u>Diabetes Care</u> 4:311, 1981.

FALLEN FOOT ARCH

CASE 29: G.E., a 57-year-old retired airline pilot, presented with a swollen left foot. Approximately 3 weeks earlier, he had had trouble putting on his left shoe. The shoe was tight and could be laced only with difficulty. Shortly thereafter, the left mid-foot appeared to be red, but the patient denied any pain, fever, or trauma to the foot. He was able to walk without difficulty. The right foot and ankle remained normal. Past medical history revealed diabetes mellitus type II for 9 years. He had been taking NPH insulin 30 U daily for the last 5 years. Other than cataracts requiring lens surgery, he attributed no complications to his diabetes.

On exam, he weighed 158 lb; height, 69 inches; BP, 135/85; pulse, 76/min and regular; temperature, 98.7°F. He was an alert male whose positive findings were: aphakia, decreased pinprick sensation bilaterally from toes to mid-calves, absent vibratory sensation over malleoli and hallux, and absent ankle and patellar deep tendon reflexes. The left mid-foot was enlarged with loss of the metatarsal arch, leaving a rocker-bottom deformity of the sole. On grasping the foot, there was crepitation and the sensation that you were holding a "bag of bones." There was no redness or skin ulceration over the feet. Excellent pedal pulses were present.

FALLEN FOOT ARCH 237

ENDOCRINE CLUE: Photograph of the feet:

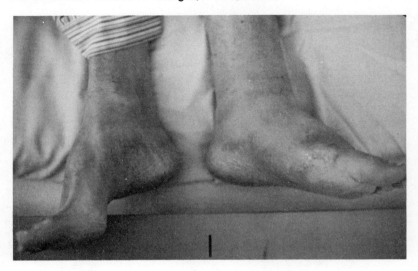

QUESTIONS:

1. What is this patient's problem?

2. Describe the "diabetic foot."

3. What findings are the result of neuropathic changes in the foot?

4. What instructions should you give the diabetic patient regarding foot care? Make a do and don't list.

5. How should this patient be managed?

6. If there should be breakdown of skin over the medial aspect of the left foot, what would you recommend?

ANSWERS:

1. <u>Charcot foot</u>. The following findings characterized the diabetic Charcot foot: **a)** peripheral neuropathy (loss of proprioception, vibratory sensation, and deep tendon reflexes); **b)** deformity (subluxation of medial tarsal leads to "rocker bottom deformity"); and **c)** good pulses, increased warmth, and swelling. The CLUE demonstrates the typical Charcot foot. Roentgenograms of this patient's foot confirm the neuropathic bone lesions. Note the changes that occurred between the previous **(A)** and current **(B)** film. The *arrow* points to subluxation of the tarsal-metarsal joints. The normal curvature of the instep is lost.

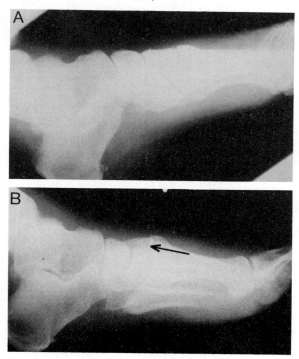

FALLEN FOOT ARCH 239

2. The <u>diabetic foot</u> represents the complications of peripheral vascular disease and neuropathy that make the foot and leg susceptible to trivial trauma, skin abrasion, callus formation, and development of ulcers that heal poorly. Often infection intervenes. Vascular disease manifests as <u>cold feet</u>, <u>absent pulses</u>, <u>blanching on elevation</u>, <u>dependent rubor</u>, <u>prolonged venous filling time</u>, <u>atrophy of subcutaneous fatty tissues</u>, <u>shiny skin</u>, <u>absent hair on foot and toes</u>, <u>thickening nails</u>, <u>infection</u>, and <u>gangrene</u>. Patients often complain of intermittent claudication and rest pain.

3. The neurological abnormalities in the diabetic foot lead to the following findings: <u>dry skin</u>, <u>painless traumas</u>, <u>atrophy of intrinsic foot muscles</u>, and <u>fragmentation of bones of the feet</u> (Charcot foot). <u>Dry skin</u> results from loss of perspiration because of autonomic dysfunction. The dry skin often cracks and fissures, leading to potential sites of infection. <u>Painless trauma</u> due to loss of sensory nerves is a major problem. Any injury may prove significant: wearing improperly fitting shoes, burns due to hot water bottles and heating pads, or trauma from foreign objects such as tacks, nails, and pebbles. <u>Atrophy of intrinsic foot muscles</u> leads to muscle weakness, causing a change in foot shape, gait, and greater pressure on skin areas prone to breakdown (e.g., hammer and claw deformity of the toes puts much more weight on metatarsal heads). <u>Charcot foot deformity</u> causes increased pressure over bony prominences, leading to ulcer formation.

4. <u>Prevention is the key to managing the diabetic foot</u>. A list of dos and don'ts provides a means of educating the patient and family. Although simple, adhering to these dos and don'ts means much in terms of hospital dollars, morbidity, and mortality.

240 CASE STUDIES IN ENDOCRINOLOGY

DOs

a) Inspect feet daily for blisters, cuts, and abrasions. If you cannot see the soles, use a mirror. If your vision is poor, get someone to check your feet.

b) Wash feet daily with lukewarm water and soap. Dry carefully, especially between the toes.

c) Apply hand cream or lanolin to dry areas of feet. Be careful not to leave cream between toes.

d) Wear clean socks or stockings daily.

e) Cut nails straight across and file down the edges with an emory board.

f) Carefully use a pumice stone or emory board to buff down any dry calluses.

g) Wear well-fitting shoes that do not rub. Make sure the shoes are comfortable before you purchase them. A wide toebox gives the toes room.

h) Wear shoes that have thick soles and that protect the toes.

i) Inspect the insides of your shoes daily for foreign objects, tacks, or torn linings.

j) Make sure your physician checks your feet at each visit.

DON'Ts

a) Do not smoke.

b) Never wash feet in hot or cold water. Check water with elbow to make sure it is lukewarm; a thermometer is even better (85-95°F).

c) Never use a heating pad, heating lamp, or hot water bottle to warm your feet.

d) Never perform bathroom surgery (razor blades, scissors) on corns and calluses. Leave that for your physician or podiatrist.

e) Avoid using any over-the-counter medications on your calluses or corns. They can cause chemical burns.

f) Do not cross your legs when sitting.

g) Do not wear garters or girdles.

h) Never go barefoot. This is especially true on beaches and around swimming pools.

i) Do not wear shoes without socks or stockings.

j) Never wear sandals with thongs between the toes.

h) Do not wear mended socks or stocking with seams.

FALLEN FOOT ARCH 241

5. <u>Make sure the patients knows the essentials of foot care listed on the previous page.</u> As long as there is considerable swelling and edema, <u>bed rest</u> is necessary. Avoid putting weight on the foot and use heel protectors since the heels of bedridden diabetic patients are particularly sensitive to pressure necrosis. Cessation of weight bearing arrests progressive destruction and promotes healing. Cast immobilization is usually not required. As clinical evidence of healing occurs, the patient is weaned from bed rest to ambulation with crutches or a walker. The affected foot must be adequately supported. Extra-depth shoes should be constructed with molding to redistribute the pressure. Metatarsal bars and arch supports do this. An insole of foam, plastic, or microcellular rubber further aids in the distribution of the weight. Shoes need high enough toe boxes to avoid the top of toes pushing against shoes.

6. Treatment of diabetic ulcer and foot infection should be prompt. <u>Bed rest</u> is imperative; <u>keep plasma glucose < 200 mg/dl</u>; <u>culture the wound</u> (pay particular attention to anaerobes); <u>begin treatment with broad-spectrum antibiotics</u> (make changes if sensitivities show more suitable antibiotics); <u>perform appropriate debridement</u> (probe sinuses, determine extent of infection); <u>X-ray for gas and bony changes</u>; <u>initiate progressive ambulation</u> with plastozote healing sandal when wound is clean and well granulated; and <u>perform surgery to remove bony prominence</u> if ulcer fails to heal. A team approach (internist, surgeon, and podiatrist) offers the best treatment for the patient.

242 CASE STUDIES IN ENDOCRINOLOGY

PEARLS:

1. The adage "an ounce of prevention is worth of a pound of cure" applies to the diabetic foot. There is a significant relationship between the development of diabetic foot lesions and the patient's understanding of foot care.

2. Infections of diabetic foot ulcers are the most frequent complication leading to hospitalization of the diabetic patient. Two-thirds of all nontraumatic amputations occur in diabetics often as result of infection.

3. Gas seen on X-ray of a diabetic foot most often means an anaerobic infection.

4. Syphilic tabes causes Charcot joints at the large joints of knee and ankle, whereas diabetes mellitus causes Charcot changes in the small joints of the foot (tarsal-metatarsal).

5. The ischemic index (systolic BP along the leg divided by the systolic BP at the antecubital fossa) helps considerably in evaluating the diabetic foot. An ischemic index < 0.5 (determined by Doppler ultrasound) warrants referral to the vascular surgeon for possible reconstructive surgery.

6. Angiography is performed only as a preoperative procedure. The criteria for doing angiography are resting or nocturnal pain not due to neuropathy; Doppler pressure at the ankle < 50% that of the arm (ischemic index < 0.5); ulcerations and infections which are not responding to bed rest, debridement, and antibiotic therapy; and gangrene or incipient gangrene of the foot.

7. There is a 90% chance for the diabetic foot ulcer to heal when the ischemic index is > 0.5. If the index is over 0.5, the basic therapeutic concept is relief of pressure over the ulcer.

FALLEN FOOT ARCH   243

8. Venous filling time (VFT) is determined by first raising the leg while the patient is supine, and then asking the patient to sit with the legs dependent (time 0). The time (seconds) that it takes any dorsal foot vein to project ever so slightly above the skin is the VFT. <u>Any patient who has VFT > 20 seconds has severely impaired circulation.</u>

PITFALLS:

1. A sad commentary is that physicians often do not inspect the feet of the diabetic patient. <u>Ask the patient to remove his or her shoes and socks.</u>

2. Too often, calluses recur because the patient is not advised about proper footwear, skin care, or maneuvers to redistribute weight.

3. The diagnosis of Charcot foot is often delayed by treating the patient for phlebitis, cellulitis, or osteomyelitis.

4. Angiography is not a totally benign procedure for the diabetic. Renal shutdown is more frequent; fortunately, the renal failure is transient and rarely permanent.

5. When culturing the diabetic ulcer, avoid getting the exudate. Material obtained deep within the tissue offers a better chance for getting the offending pathogen. Do not forget to get anaerobic cultures as well.

6. In treating the diabetic ulcer, <u>soaks are rarely indicated.</u> Soaking leads to macerated tissue and promotes further spread of bacteria.

244 CASE STUDIES IN ENDOCRINOLOGY

7. Determing venous filling time is useless in patients with varicose veins.

REFERENCES

Delbridge L, Appleberg M, Reeve TS: Factors associated with development of foot lesions in the diabetic. Surgery 93:78, 1983.

Gleckman RA, Roth RM: Diabetic foot infections—prevention and treatment. West J Med 142:263, 1985.

Levin ME: The diabetic foot. Angiology 31:375, 1980.

Wagner FW Jr: The treatment of the diabetic foot. Compr Ther 10:29, 1984.

White RR IV, Lynch DJ, Verheyen CN, et al: Management of the wounds in the diabetic foot. Surg Clin North Am 64:735, 1984.

DIABETES MELLITUS AND SURGERY

CASE 30: D.P., a 54-year-old automobile mechanic, is admitted for an elective cholecystectomy. Eight weeks previously he had right upper quadrant pain associated with fever, leukocytosis, and elevated serum alkaline phosphatase. An oral cholecystogram failed to visualize the gall bladder. Sonograms confirmed gallstones. He has had diabetes mellitus for 15 years and takes 40 U of NPH insulin each morning. He reportedly follows a 2200-calorie diet each day but has been unsuccessful in losing weight. The only known complication of diabetes is early bilateral cataracts. Family history is positive for diabetes mellitus (mother and maternal uncle).

On examination, he weighed 169 lb; height, 69 inches; BP, 130/85; pulse, 65/min and regular; and temperature, 98.7°F. A few lenticular opacities were present, but not enough to obscure the fundus (see CLUE). Over the mid-anterior thighs, there were several nontender, depressed areas that represented loss of subcutaneous fat. No ankle jerks could be elicited. The remainder of the exam was normal.

ENDOCRINE CLUE:

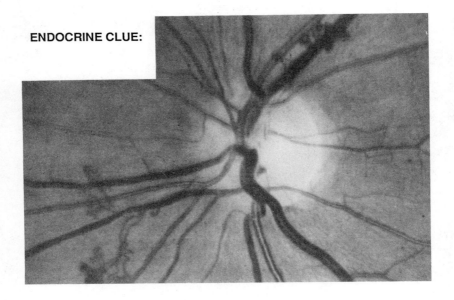

QUESTIONS:

1. What findings do you note in the CLUE?

2. What are the depressed areas over the thighs?

3. What goals should you have for managing this patient for his surgery?

4. How can you meet these goals?

5. What are the specific orders that you write on his chart?

248   CASE STUDIES IN ENDOCRINOLOGY

ANSWERS:

1. <u>Diabetic proliferative retinopathy</u>. Note the tufts of frond-like vessels within a disk diameter of the optic disk at the 1 and 7 o'clock positions. This represents neovascularization. These vessels proliferate in response to ischemia and are most often seen near the disk margins. These new vessels lack mural pericytes for support, making them subject to rupture. Hemorrhage into the retina and vitreous with resultant scarring leads to blindness. This patient needs an ophthalmology consultation for treatment of his retinopathy. Pan-retinal photocoagulation decreases oxygen requirements throughout the retina and thus retards the neovascular process.

2. <u>Diabetic lipoatrophy</u>. Loss of fat at sites of previous insulin injections is due to a reaction involving immune complex formation with less purified insulins of bygone days. One sees lipoatrophy much less frequently since purer insulin preparations have been introduced. Lipoatrophy usually resolves within 6-9 months after changing to highly purified insulin which is injected into the periphery of the depressed areas.

3. Goals: **a)** <u>Good preoperative control</u>. Control of the diabetes will make elective surgery and anesthesia management much easier. Uncontrolled diabetes coupled with the stress of surgery may progress to ketoacidosis or hyperosmolar coma. **b)** <u>Keep the patient from having hyperglycemia</u> (plasma glucoses > 200 mg/dl), which impairs wound healing and increases susceptibility to infection. **c)** <u>Avoid hypoglycemia</u>.

4. <u>There are a number of methods to cover the diabetic who needs general surgery</u>. It is important, regardless of the regimen used, that the patient's blood sugars be monitored frequently. Fingerstick blood glucose, recorded at the

DIABETES MELLITUS AND SURGERY   249

bedside, is rapid and convenient. The frequency of blood glucose checks must to be individualized. Most patients are kept fasting after midnight prior to surgery. An intravenous 5% dextrose solution, 100-150 ml/hour, is started around dawn and regular insulin is given subcutaneously. The amount and route of insulin administration depend on the patient's normal total daily insulin dose and the type of surgery. The total daily dose is divided by 4. This value is given as regular insulin subcutaneously every 6 hours as long as intravenous fluids are being infused. The first dose is usually given at 7-8 AM on the day of surgery. This regimen is used for all surgery except those operations requiring hypothermia (e.g., cardiac), where absorption may be erratic. In these special situations, regular insulin is given as a continuous intravenous drip at 1-2 U/hour. The rate is increased or decreased according to fingerstick blood glucose levels. Blood sugars between 100-200 mg/dl are acceptable.

Postoperatively, a better regimen than the "sliding scale" is to maintain the every-6-hour insulin program and supplement the doses with additional regular insulin in amounts based on the plasma glucose. Additional regular insulin is added to the every-6-hour insulin regimen by using an algorithm based on the blood sugar just prior to the scheduled injection (the advantage of fingersticks and reflectometer readings at bedside is obvious). For blood sugars between 200 and 249 mg/dl, add 2-4 U; for blood sugars between 250 and 299 mg/dl, add 3-6 U; and for blood sugars > 300 mg/dl, add 5-10 U. Using the rule of 5% of the total daily dose for each 50 mg/dl above 200 mg/dl for supplements is helpful. Double the supplements for moderate or large ketosis (unless the ketosis is due to starvation when the plasma glucoses are reasonable). The exact extra amount varies depending on the basal dose, with the larger amounts being used for patients receiving larger basal doses. If the basal amount needs constant supplementation, then the basal dose is raised; if

250 CASE STUDIES IN ENDOCRINOLOGY

the blood sugar is low (< 60 mg/dl), then the basal dose is reduced. <u>Insulin orders generally require rewriting once or twice daily.</u>

As soon as the patient can eat, regular insulin is given before meals and before bedtime with a bedtime snack. The <u>same</u> dose of regular insulin should <u>not</u> be given before meals and at bedtime because of the overlap of insulin effect with the breakfast dose at 0800 and the lunch dose at 1200, etc. Once the patient can eat, administer the total daily dose of regular insulin as follows: 1/3 before breakfast, 1/6 before lunch, 1/3 before supper, and 1/6 at bedtime. No more than 10 U is given at bedtime (hs), and supplements are not added to the hs dose to avoid nocturnal hypoglycemia. Alternatively, the preoperative program may be reinstituted and regular insulin added for anteprandial blood sugars > 200 mg/dl. <u>The importance of monitoring the sugar and making day-to-day adjustments can not be overemphasized.</u>

5. These orders are written for control of diabetes and do not take into account other parameters such as electrolyte check and pre- and postoperative medications.

   a) For OR in AM; NPO p midnight.
   b) IV D5W at 125 ml/hour to begin at 0600.
   c) D/C current insulin orders.
   d) Begin regular insulin U-100 <u>10 U sc q 6 hours at 0700</u> (basal regimen).
   e) Check blood glucose by reflectometer q 6 hours while on ward (begin at 0650), and hourly while in OR and recovery room. If question of hypoglycemia, check PRN. <u>Record sugars on flow sheet.</u>
   f) Add regular insulin supplements to the basal regimen (10 U q 6 hours) <u>if</u> blood sugars are > 200 mg/dl. For values 200-249 mg/dl, add 2 U of regular insulin; for values 250-299 mg/dl, add 4 U of regular insulin; for values 300-400

DIABETES MELLITUS AND SURGERY 251

mg/dl, add 6 U of regular insulin; for values > 400 mg/dl, call HO.

g) Postoperatively, continue qid regular insulin as long as IVs are running.

h) NPO until nausea passes. Begin clear liquids and progress to regular diabetic diet as patient tolerates. Bring tray at 0700, 1200, 1800, and 2300 hours.

j) Continue qid blood glucose checks and supplemental insulin program.

i) When able to eat home diet program, discontinue IVs and supplemental hs (2300 hour) insulin program.

k) Return to home program of 40 U NPH q AM 30-45 minutes ac breakfast. Give regular insulin 10 U along with 40 U NPH on the first day when starting NPH (will need regular insulin to carryover to first day of NPH after being on qid regular schedule). Add supplements if needed before meals only (not at hs).

l) Make sure the nutritionist or dietician sees the patient to make recommendations.

PEARLS:

1. Repeated injection into the same area cause lipohypertrophy ("insulin tumors"). Frequent rotation of the injection sites avoids this problem.

2. A flow sheet that records all glucose and insulin data is essential to interpret patterns and to write appropriate insulin orders.

3. Scheduling the diabetic patient first for the OR in the morning facilitates management.

252 CASE STUDIES IN ENDOCRINOLOGY

PITFALLS:

1. All intravenous fluids given to the postoperative insulin-treated patients should contain 5% glucose.

2. Postoperative orders using urine glucose for "a sliding-scale insulin" dose are a surgical tradition but should be avoided. Since the renal threshold for glucose must be exceeded before any glycosuria is detected, the "sliding scale" treats hyperglycemia after the fact, and does not offer a means of preventing hyperglycemia.

3. Never write a <u>routine</u> supplemental insulin order for bedtime. A sleeping patient and a lean ward staff on the "graveyard" shift make detecting hypoglycemia difficult.

REFERENCES

Gallina DL, Mordes JP, Rossini AA: Surgery in the diabetic patient. <u>Compr Ther</u> 9:8, 1983.

George K, Alberti MM, Gill GV, et al: Insulin delivery during surgery in the diabetic patient. <u>Diabetes Care</u> 5 (Suppl 1):65, 1982.

McMurry JR Jr: Wound healing with diabetes mellitus: better glucose control for better wound healing in diabetes. <u>Surg Clin North Am</u> 64:769, 1984.

Podolsky S: Management of diabetes in the surgical patient. <u>Med Clin North Am</u> 66:1361, 1982.

Shuman CR: Surgery in the diabetic patient. <u>Compr Ther</u> 8:38, 1982.

Thomas DJB, Hinds CJ, Rees GM: The management of insulin dependent diabetes during cardiopulmonary bypass and general surgery. <u>Anaesthesia</u> 38:1047, 1983.

SHOW AND TELL

CASE 31: R.R., a 32-year-old attorney, was found to have a serum calcium of 8.3 mg/dl on routine screening chemistries. He had no specific complaints. On examination he was 64 inches tall and was moderately overweight (160 lb). A photograph and X-ray of his hand are given below. What is the diagnosis?

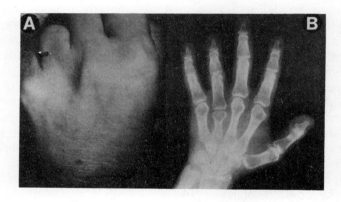

254   CASE STUDIES IN ENDOCRINOLOGY

ANSWER:

The combination of a low serum calcium and a "dimple" over the knuckles (**A**) due to a short metacarpal (**B**) is characteristic of pseudohypoparathyroidism (PHP). PHP is a familial syndrome of hypocalcemia associated with raised levels of PTH and resistance to PTH action. A characteristic physiognomy (Albright's osteodystrophy) of round facies, short stature, and short metacarpals and metatarsals (fourth and fifth digits) is present in the classic syndrome. The importance of this syndrome relates not to its frequency but rather to its contribution to our understanding of the pathophysiology of hormone resistance in general. PHP is managed as hypoparathyroidism but is often easier to treat than idiopathic hypoparathyroidism, probably because the hormone resistance is not total. Patients who have the stigmata of Albright's osteodystrophy (short stature, obesity, and dystrophic bone changes) without hypocalcemia are said to have pseudo-pseudohypoparathyroidism (PPHP). PPHP is genetically related to but distinct from PHP.

SHOW AND TELL   255

CASE 32: L.S., a 29-year-old stockbroker, was admitted to the ward for evaluation of palpitations and intermittent tachycardia. The attending physician asked that a TRH study be performed. What is TRH? How would you write the orders? How would you interpret the results of this study given below?

Serum thyroid-stimulating hormone (TSH) at 0 time: 3.0 µU/ml; TSH at 30 minutes: 16 µU/ml.

256   CASE STUDIES IN ENDOCRINOLOGY

ANSWERS:

Thyrotropin-releasing hormone (TRH) is a tripeptide secreted by the hypothalamus and circulated to the pituitary via the portal-hypophyseal capillary system. TRH stimulates pituitary thyrotropes to secrete TSH (thyrotropin). If ambient levels of T4 or T3 are high, then the thyrotrope will not respond to TRH with a rise in TSH. In primary hypothyroidism, the TSH is already elevated; TRH greatly augments the release of TSH. TRH administration is extremely useful clinically in states in which hyperthyroidism is suspected and the diagnosis is not clear using static determinations such as T4(RIA), T3U, and T3(RIA). Giving TRH provides a dynamic test which assesses the functional integrity of the thyrotrope.

The TRH study is performed as follows: Blood is drawn for baseline TSH (0 time). TRH (protirelin) 500 µg is given intravenously over 15-20 seconds and blood is drawn again at 30 minutes for TSH determination. TSH levels peak normally around 20-30 minutes post TRH infusion.

The normal response is dependent upon age and sex. Females generally have at least a 6 µU/ml rise above the basal level. Males < 40 years of age should have a similar rise (> 6 µU/ml), whereas males > 40 years should have at least a 2 µU/ml rise. In primary hypothyroidism, the response to TRH is exaggerated. Hyperthyroid patients, patients with euthyroid Graves' disease, or subjects taking excessive doses of replacement thyroid (T4 or T3) or pharmacological amounts of glucocorticoid will not have a rise in serum TSH. In patients suspected of having hyperthyroidism, the TRH study has nearly replaced the use of exogenous thyroid hormone to see whether radioiodine uptake is suppressed or not.

This patient's TRH study was normal, thus excluding hyperthyroidism as a cause of the tachycardia.

SHOW AND TELL 257

CASE 33: D.H., a 60-year-old widow, has had a long history of recurrent nephrolithiasis. What does the photograph show? What is its implication?

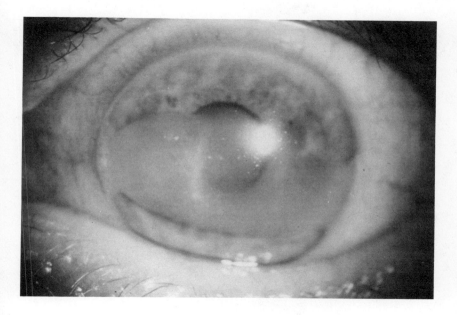

258   CASE STUDIES IN ENDOCRINOLOGY

ANSWERS:

The photograph demonstrates classic band keratopathy. Note the cloudy band extending across the cornea that represents calcium deposition within the cornea. Band keratopathy indicates hypercalcemia of long duration (see pages 188-192). A serum calcium should be obtained.

CASE 34: P.W., a 32-year-old housewife, presented with a 2.5-cm firm mass in the anterior triangle on the left side of the neck. A photograph of this patient is given below. What is the diagnosis?

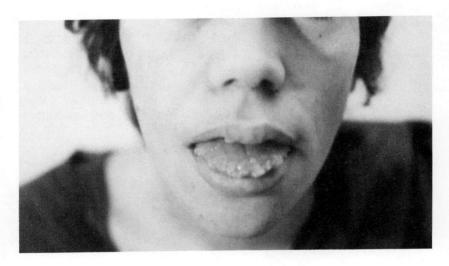

ANSWER:

The photograph shows multiple nodular lesions on the edge of the tongue. On close examination these nodules are firm and light yellow in color. These mucosal neuromas are characteristic of patients who have multiple endocrine neoplasia type IIb. The mass in her neck was metastatic medullary thyroid carcinoma. Case 10 (pages 72-78) discusses this problem. The familial nature of this disorder is emphasized in the following photograph of this patient's daughter, who already had elevated plasma calcitonin levels and medullary thyroid carcinoma at the age of 6 years.

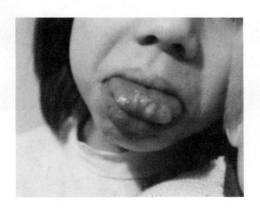

CASE 35: Shown are photographs of two patients who share the same problem. What is the diagnosis?

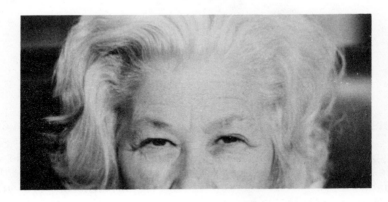

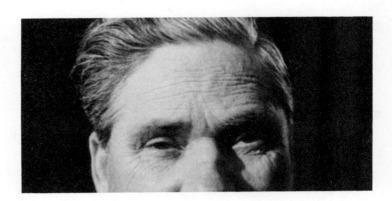

262 CASE STUDIES IN ENDOCRINOLOGY

ANSWER:

Hypothyroidism is most likely. Note the similar appearance of the upper eyelids. Also compare with the photograph of Case 14 (page 101). Of course, these facial features are not pathognomonic of hypothyroidism. Similar changes may be found in normal individuals and some patients with hypopituitarism.

SHOW AND TELL 263

Case 36: Photograph of the hands of a 50-year-old school teacher. What is the most likely diagnosis?

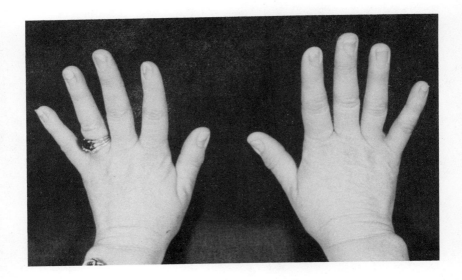

264 CASE STUDIES IN ENDOCRINOLOGY

ANSWER:

The fingernails show impressive onycholysis. Though trauma at the edge of the nailbed often causes onycholysis, this degree of onycholysis is diagnostic of <u>hyperthyroidism</u>. These nails may be called "Plummer's nails."

CASE 37: J.R., a 68-year-old retired saleman, had been in excellent health until he was admitted to the hospital for the evaluation of progressive confusion and mental deterioration. He was taking no medications. The physical exam was unremarkable. Serum studies on admission: glucose, 98 mg/dl; Na, 124 mEq/l; Cl, 89 mEq/l; HCO_3, 20 mEq/dl; Ca, 9.0 mg/dl. Urine specific gravity: 1.014. His chest X-ray is shown below. What is the most likely diagnosis?

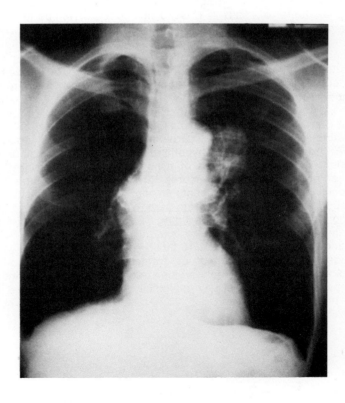

266   CASE STUDIES IN ENDOCRINOLOGY

ANSWER:

Syndrome of inappropriate ADH secretion secondary to bronchogenic carcinoma (note the chest X-ray shows a mass in the left lung). Antidiuretic hormone secretion in the presence of low plasma osmolality and in the absence of physiologic states that cause ADH secretion (e.g., dehydration, hypovolemia, or hypotension) characterizes the syndrome of inappropriate antidiuretic hormone (SIADH). Continual ADH secretion leads to water retention and dilutional hyponatremia. The diagnosis of SIADH should be suspected when there is a combination of hyponatremia (serum sodium usually < 130 mEq/l) and an inappropriately concentrated urine. The urine sodium is usually > 20 mEq/l in SIADH patients who are taking normal amounts of salt. This is in contrast to patients with hyponatremia with decreased effective blood volume (e.g., heart failure, ascites) where renal tubular resorption of sodium is increased and the urine sodium is < 20 mEq/l. There are multiple causes of SIADH: 1) ectopic production of ADH (SIADH was first described in patients with bronchogenic carcinoma, which remains the most common cause of this syndrome); 2) central nervous system disorders (head injuries, vascular lesions, infections, Guillain-Barre syndrome, and acute intermittent porphyria); 3) drugs (vincristine, chlorpropamide, carbamazepine); and 4) endocrine disease (Addison's disease, hypothyroidism). The clinical features are weight gain and symptoms of hyponatremia (weakness, lethargy, and mental confusion). Seizures are treated with intravenous hypertonic saline (5%) in amounts to increase the serum sodium to 120 mEq/l. All SIADH patients are volume replete and need restriction of fluids to < 1000 ml/day. Sodium loading is not helpful since these patients respond by excreting it into the urine without correcting the hyponatremia. If fluid restriction does not work or the underlying disorder cannot be treated effectively (e.g., oat cell carcinoma of the lung), then administration of demeclocycline 300 mg three to four times a day to inhibit ADH's action on the renal tubule may prove effective.

SHOW AND TELL   267

CASE 38: A 58-year-old house painter was admitted to the hospital with sepsis and aspiration pneumonia. Although the patient had no goiter or skin findings of thyroid disease, thyroid function studies were ordered because of lethargy and apparent dementia. The following levels were obtained: T4(RIA), 4.0 µg/dl (normal, 5-12); T3U, 35% (normal, 35-45); free thyroid index, 1.6 (normal, 2.2-4.7); T3(RIA), 70 ng/dl (normal, 90-180). Later, a serum TSH level was ordered: TSH, 1.0 µU/ml. What is this patient's diagnosis?

268   CASE STUDIES IN ENDOCRINOLOGY

ANSWER:

In this setting, one relies heavily on the serum TSH. If there is no clinical evidence of pituitary dysfunction, then euthyroid sick is the most likely diagnosis. Euthyroid sick is a term designated for those patients with nonthyroidal illnesses who have abnormal thyroid tests. The results can be classified into the following categories: 1) low T3 syndrome; 2) low T3 and low T4 syndrome; 3) high T4 syndrome; and 4) a mixed form in which a combination of abnormalites may be found.

Low T3 syndrome is the most common of the euthyroid sick abnormalities, but it is usually not identified since most screening studies do not measure T3(RIA). The serum T3(RIA) is low and the serum T4(RIA) is normal. The patient is clinically euthyroid. The serum T3(RIA) may be low in many circumstances: systemic illnesses (e.g., liver disease, acute febrile illnesses, renal failure, neoplastic disorders, burns, and congestive heart failure); starvation; major surgery; and following the administration of some drugs (dexamethasone, cholecystographic dyes, amiodarone, high doses of propranolol, and thionamides). The common factor in all these conditions is reduced extrathyroidal conversion of T4 to T3. The conversion of reverse T3 (rT3) to T2 is impaired, leading to increased levels of serum rT3. The TSH is normal, and the free T4 measured by dialysis techniques is normal or high. The low T3 resolves when the underlying illness clears.

This patient fits into the low T3 and low T4 syndrome, which is usually identified because a low serum T4(RIA) found on screening for thyroid disease. The free thyroid index (FTI) is often low as well. These patients are severely ill and the clinical assessment to totally exclude hypothyroidism is difficult. However, careful history and physical examination will not reveal the typical features of hypothyroidism. Free T4 levels are low, normal, or high. Serum TSH and TRH testing (i.e., TSH response to TRH) are normal. Patients who have a low T3 and low T4 generally do not do well when the T4(RIA) is < 3 µg/dl (mortality approaches 84%) and underscores the severity of the nonthyroidal illness found in this set of patients. There no evidence that treatment with L-thyroxine helps these patients.

SHOW AND TELL   269

CASE 39: C.D., a 58-year-old fisherman, was found to have Cushingoid features by his personal physician. Baseline urine studies confirmed hypercortisolism. A CT scan of the adrenals was interpreted as normal. In addition to the dexamethasone studies (pages 5-6), the attending endocrinologist asks for a metyrapone study. What is the rationale for ordering this test? What do you write on the order sheet?

ANSWERS:

Metyrapone inhibits the final enzymatic step (11-beta-hydroxylase) in the synthesis of cortisol. This leads to a build-up of 11-deoxycortisol, the immediate precursor of cortisol, and to a decrease in cortisol production. The fall in serum cortisol levels is sensed by the pituitary corticotrophs, which respond by increasing ACTH production in the classical negative feedback loop. Although serum deoxycortisol levels rise, the pituitary does not recognize deoxycortisol as a glucocorticoid hormone. As a result, in normal subjects administration of metyrapone leads to elevated levels of deoxycortisol and low, normal, or raised serum cortisol (the absolute levels of cortisol depend upon the effectiveness of the metyrapone-induced blockade). In patients with pituitary insufficiency or in patients with Cushing's syndrome due to ectopic ACTH production (pages 38-40) or due to an adrenal adenoma/carcinoma, plasma deoxycortisol fails to rise in response to metyrapone loading. In Cushing's disease (pituitary-dependent adrenal hyperplasia), there is an exaggerated response, leading to high levels of deoxycortisol. So, administering metyrapone to this patient could provide helpful information as to the etiology of the hypercortisolism.

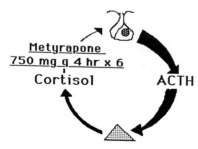 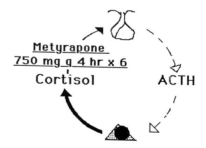

SHOW AND TELL 271

Metyrapone is usually administrated orally using either of the two following protocols: an abbreviated overnight study which is used mainly to evaluate for pituitary insufficiency or the classic 3-day study used to assess the pituitary-adrenal axis. This patient needs the latter study.

Urine is collected for 24 hours as a baseline for determination of 17-OHCS (day 1). Metyrapone is given 750 mg every 4 hours by mouth for 6 doses (day 2). Since both cortisol and deoxycortisol have the 17,21-dihydroxyl,20-keto groups which are measured in the Porter-Silber reaction of the 17-OHCS assay, urine 17-OHCS levels normally rise. A 24-hour urine is collected on day 3 (the day following oral metyrapone). A normal rise in urine 17-OHCS is 2.5 to 3 times the baseline day's 17-OHCS value. 17-OHCS is measured on the day after metyrapone dosage since the last two doses of metyrapone given on day 2 produce the lowest cortisol levels (early morning), which stimulate ACTH and thus steroidogenesis, which is reflected in the large amount of 17-OHCS in the subsequent collection. Patients with Cushing's disease increase their urine 17-OHCS > fourfold over baseline. Patients with adrenal tumors fail to increase 17-OHCS in response to metyrapone loading.

Levels of plasma cortisol and deoxycortisol at 7-8 AM on days 2 and 3 following metyrapone dosage are necessary to assess the adequacy of the metyrapone blockade. Furthermore, plasma deoxycortisol levels are helpful in defining the etiology of the hypercortisolism. Patients with Cushing's disease should have post metyrapone 11-deoxycortisol levels (0700 hours on day 3) that are > 10 μg/dl. Patients with adrenocortical neoplasm have suppressed 11-deoxycortisol levels (< 10 μg/dl). Sample protocol orders for this study are given on the next page.

272 CASE STUDIES IN ENDOCRINOLOGY

Orders for metyrapone loading study:

1) **DAY 1:** Collect 24-hour urine (0700 to 0700 hours) for 17-OHCS.

2) **DAY 2:** Blood draw at 0700 for plasma cortisol and deoxycortisol.

Administer metyrapone 750 mg q 4 hours po times 6 doses (Start giving medication at 0800 hours).

Collect 24-hour urine (0700 to 0700 hours) for 17-OHCS.

3) **DAY 3:** Blood draw at 0700 for plasma cortisol and deoxycortisol.

Collect 24-hour urine (0700 to 0700 hours) for 17-OHCS.

CASE 40: R. J., a 42-year-old machinist, presents for evaluation of profuse perspiration, frequent headaches, and newly diagnosed hypertension. On examination his physiognomy and body features were abnormal. You note multiple skin lesions. The photograph of this patient's right axilla demonstrates these lesions. What is the diagnosis?

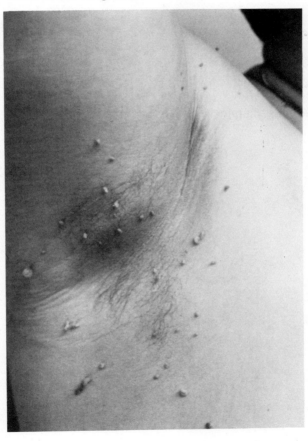

274 CASE STUDIES IN ENDOCRINOLOGY

ANSWER:

The photograph shows multiple skin tags that are often seen in acromegaly. The history is also suggestive of acromegaly. The remainder of the exam and his growth hormone studies confirmed this diagnosis (pages 116-120).

CASE 41: T.G., a 35-year-old clerk-typist, had a 1-cm nonsecreting pituitary adenoma removed by transsphenoidal pituitary microsurgery 6 weeks ago. She presents for follow-up evaluation of her pituitary status. She has not been on any medications. You are asked to write the orders to evaluate this patient for hypopituitarism. What studies would you order? How would you interpret the results of her studies given below?

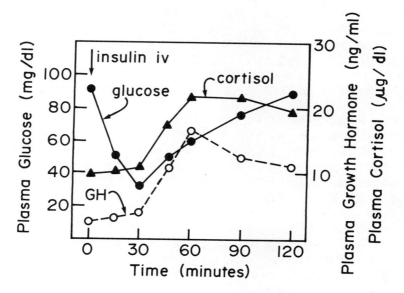

Response of plasma growth hormone and plasma cortisol to insulin-induced hypoglycemia.

276 CASE STUDIES IN ENDOCRINOLOGY

ANSWERS:

Evaluation for pituitary hypofunction entails both static and dynamic studies. Static studies are single serum or urine samples that assess baseline function. Such studies include T4(RIA) and T3U (to evaluate thyroid function), urine specific gravity (to assess ADH), or 24-hour urine for free cortisol (to indirectly evaluate ACTH). However, dynamic or provocative studies often test the adequacy or reserve for several tropic hormones. The "gold standard" dynamic study is insulin-induced hypoglycemia. Hypoglycemia produces a profound stress reaction that is followed by growth hormone (GH) and ACTH release with a subsequent rise in the serum cortisol. The insulin-induced hypoglycemia test (IIHT) is an excellent method to gather GH and cortisol data to assess the integrity of the pituitary-adrenal axis.

The insulin-induced hypoglycemia test is performed in the morning after an overnight fast with the patient at bed rest. An indwelling needle in the forearm is recommended so that multiple samples can be obtained. Blood for basal levels of GH and cortisol is taken at -15 and 0 minutes. Regular insulin (0.1 U/kg for normal-weight patients and 0.15-0.2 U/kg for patients with insulin resistance, e.g., obesity) is rapidly injected intravenously. If there is clinical evidence of hypopituitarism, then a lower dose of insulin is used (0.05 U/kg) since profound hypoglycemia is more likely. Plasma glucose is measured at 0, 15, 30, 45, and 60 minutes. A decrease of the plasma glucose to 50% of baseline value or < 40 mg/dl is considered an adequate hypoglycemic response, which is necessary to interpret the GH and cortisol levels. Blood for GH and cortisol is measured at 0, 30, 60, and 90 minutes. Dextrose (50%) should be available to treat severe hypoglycemia (e.g. obtundation, seizure). After hypoglycemia is assured (hunger, palpitations, perspiration), the patient may drink fruit juice to decrease symptoms if necessary. The nadir for the blood sugar is usually 20-30 minutes into the study with rises of GH and cortisol later. Even though sugar may have to be given intravenously or by mouth, continue to draw blood at the indicated intervals.

GH levels normally rise to > 9 ng/ml 60-90 minutes post insulin injection. Plasma cortisol should rise at least 10 µg/dl to a value > 20 µg/dl in normal subjects. This patient had a normal response to insulin-induced hypoglycemia. The IIHT assumes the adrenal glands can function to respond to ACTH. Since hypoglycemia is potentially life threatening to the hypoadrenal patient, one should avoid this study in patients with known Addison's disease. The disadvantages of insulin-induced hypoglycemia are obvious: close monitoring of the patient is a necessity; hypoglycemia is uncomfortable and potential problems are very real; it is not easily performed in children; and one must be sure of adequate hypoglycemia (stress) to have a valid study. In addition, up to 20% of normal subjects have an impaired or absent GH response to this "gold standard." Patients with obesity, Cushing's syndrome, and chronic renal failure may also have an impaired or absent GH response. However, a normal response excludes GH deficiency.

Index

Acetest, 216
Acetoacetate, 216
Acetone, 210, 216
Acromegaloidism, 116, 118
Acromegaly, 114-121
  diagnosis, 116
  treatment, 117
ACTH (see Adrenocorticotropic
  hormone)
Addison's disease, 44-48
  chronic treatment of, 45-46
  diagnosis, 44-45
Adenomatosis, multiple endocrine,
  (see Multiple endocrine neoplasia)
ADH (see Antidiuretic hormone)
Adrenal:
  adrenal adenomas, 12-21
  androgens, 152, 156
  carcinoma, 5-7, 10, 156
  Cushing's syndrome, 1-11, 36-41, 155
  hypofunction,
    (see Addison's disease)
  tests for, 25, 44-45
  treatment of, 44-45
  incidental mass, 21-28
Adrenocorticotropic hormone (ACTH), 4-7,
  10
  Addison's disease, 44
  Cushing's disease, 1-11
  deficiency, 108-113, 269
  ectopic production and, 34-41
  handling of specimen, 9
  metyrapone, 270-271
  stimulation tests, 270-271
  suppression tests, 4-6
Albright's osteodystrophy, 253-254
Alcohol:
  hypoglycemia and, 174

Aldosterone:
  deficiency, 44-46
  excess, 12-20
  measurement, 14-15
  potassium and, 14, 18
  renin and, 15, 19
Alkaline phosphatase activity:
  hyperparathyroidism, 193-194
  osteomalacia and, 181
  osteoporosis, 204
Amenorrhea, 1, 149, 159
  evaluation (flow diagram), 165
  galactorrhea and, 122
  gonadal dysgenesis and, 166
  treatment, 166
Amiodarone, 88, 268
Androgens:
  adrenal, 152, 156
  deficiency, 143
  excess, 149-158
  resistance to, 162-163, 167
Androstenedione, 152-153
Anorexia nervosa, 162
Anticonvulsants, 183
Antidiuretic hormone, 129-138
  deficiency, 132
  dehydration test and, 133
  diabetes insipidus and, 129-138
  inappropriate secretion (SIADH), 266
  replacement therapy, 135
Antithyroid drugs, 83-84, 90
Asherman's syndrome, 164, 166
Autoimmune endocrine disease:
  Addison's disease and, 44
  diabetes mellitus and, 218
  Hashimoto's thyroiditis, 69, 102, 105-106
  hyperthyroidism, 82
  hypothyroidism, 100-107

279

280 INDEX

Band keratopathy, 185-186, 257-258
Body weight, ideal, 221
Breast:
  galactorrhea and, 122-128
Bromocriptine, 126-127, 144

C-peptide, 173
Calciferol (see Ergocalciferol)
Calcifediol (see 25-hydroxyvitamin D)
Calcitriol (see 1,25-dihydroxyvitamin D)
Calcitonin:
  medullary thyroid carcinoma, 72-78
  pentagastrin and, 75
Calcium:
  deficiency (see Hypocalcemia)
  excess (see Hypercalcemia)
  hypercalciuria, 125-126
  multiple endocrine neoplasia, 34, 75, 191
  supplementation (table), 182
Catecholamines:
  hypoglycemia and, 170
  measurement of, 32
  tumor production, 27-35
Chlorpropamide, 135, 173, 224
Choriocarcinoma, 82
Chvostek's sign, 180, 184
Clomiphene, 154
Cortisol:
  deficiency, 42-48
  hypoglycemia and, 275, 277
  metyrapone and, 270-271
  plasma levels, 28
  replacement therapy, 45
  suppression tests, 2, 8-9
  urine levels, 4-6, 44
Cortisone acetate, 45
Cosyntropin study, 44, 156
Cushing's disease, 1-12
Cushing's syndrome, 1-12, 25, 36-41
  causes, 5
  dexamethasone suppression and, 5-6
  ectopic ACTH and, 36-41
  iatrogenic, 8
  tests for, 4-7
Cyproterone acetate, 154

Dawn phenomenon, 233
DDAVP, 135, 137
Dehydroepiandrosterone (DHEA),152, 156
11-Deoxycortisol, 270-271
Dexamethasone:

suppression test, 4-6
Diabetes insipidus:
  causes, 132
  diagnosis, 129
  nephrogenic, 137
  neurogenic, 129-138
  treatment, 135
  triphasic response, 137
Diabetes mellitus, 207-252
  classification, 218
  complications, 213, 226, 228, 236
  diagnosis, 210, 220
  diet and, 220-221
  exercise and, 220
  glucose tolerance test and, 220, 223-224
  glycosylated hemoglobin, 224, 228
  insulin therapy, 211-212, 230-232, 249-250
  ketoacidosis, 207
  management, 220-224, 229-234, 240-243
  mucormycosis, 213-214
  neuropathy and, 237-239
  retinopathy and, 245, 248
  sulfonylureas and, 222-224
  surgery and, 245-252
Diazoxide, 172
Diet:
  diabetes mellitus and, 220-221
  hypoglycemia and, 175
Dihydrotachysterol, 182
Dihydrotestosterone, 153, 156
1,25-dihydroxyvitamin D:
  hypocalcemia and, 182
  osteomalacia and, 181
  treatment with, 182

Ectopic hormone syndromes:
  antidiuretic hormone (ADH), 265-266
  adenocorticotropic hormone (ACTH), 36-41
Ergocalciferol:
  for hypocalcemia, 182
Estrogens:
  amenorrhea and, 162, 166
  osteoporosis and, 201, 203-204
  treatment:
    for hyperparathyroidism, 192
    for hypogonadism,166
    for osteoporosis, 204
Euthyroid sick, 60, 267-268
Exophthalmos, 89

INDEX 281

Eye:
diabetes mellitus and, 228, 245, 248
pituitary tumors and, 108-113
thyroid disease and, 82, 89

Familial dysalbuminemic hyperthyroxinemia,
60-61
Fasting:
glucose, 170, 220
growth hormone, 116, 118
hypoglycemia, 168-176
Fine needle aspiration biopsy, 27, 65-67, 74
Fludocortisone, 46
Follicule stimulating hormone (FSH),
152-153, 166
Foot ulcers, diabetic, 241-243
Fructose intolerance, 171
Functional hypoglycemia, 175
Functional impotence, 144-146

Galactorrhea, 122-128
Gastric surgery, and
hypocalcemia, 177, 180
GH (see Growth hormone)

Globulin:
sex-binding, 157
thyroid-binding, 58-59
Glucagon, 174
Glucose:
acromegaly and, 106
hyperglycemia
(see Diabetes mellitus)
hypoglycemia, 168-176
plasma levels, 170
tolerance tests:
glucose, 220
insulin-induced, 275-277
Glycohemoglobin, 224, 228
Glycyrrhizinic acid, 17
Goiter:
diffuse toxic, 79-85
nodular, 93-99
pseudogoiter, 52-55
simple, 52
toxic multinodular, 86-92
Gonadal dysgenesis, 145, 162, 166
Gonadotropins:
amenorrhea and, 163
chorionic, 164

follicule stimulating hormone, 152-153,
166
luteinizing hormone, 145, 163, 166
Gonads (see Hypogonadism, Ovaries, or
Testes)
Granulomatous diseases:
adrenal, 50
diabetes insipidus and, 134
hypercalcemia and, 126
thyroid and, 52, 69, 105-106
Graves' disease (see
Hyperthyroidism)
clinical features, 79, 82
therapy of, 83-84
Growth hormone:
acromegaly, 114-116
deficiency, 113, 275-277
insulin-induced hypoglycemia, 275-277
reserve, 275-277
suppression with glucose, 116-117
TRH study, 118

Hashimoto's thyroiditis, 52, 69, 105-106
Hemochromatosis, 44, 46, 146
Hirsutism, 149-158
therapy, 154
H-Y antigen, 166
Hydrocortisone (see Cortisol)
Hydroxybutyrate, 215
17-Hydroxycorticoids, urine, 4-10, 271
21-Hydroxylase, 156
17-Hydroxyprogesterone, 156
Hyperaldosteronism (see Aldosterone)
Hypercalcemia, 186-196
Addison's disease and, 47
differential diagnosis (table), 189
familial hypocalciuric, 195
hyperparathyroidism and, 188-190
immobilization and, 179
malignancy and, 188-190
multiple endocrine neoplasia, 34, 75, 194
parathyroid carcinoma, 193
thiazide-related, 190
therapy for, 191-192
vitamin D intoxication, 126
vitamin A intoxication, 126
Hypercortisolism (see Cushing's
syndrome)
Hyperglycemia (see Diabetes mellitus)
Hyperinsulinism (see Hypoglycemia)

282 INDEX

Hyperkalemia:
 Addison's disease and, 44-45
 ketoacidosis and, 212
Hyperparathyroidism, 186-196
 diagnosis, 188
 primary, 186-189
 therapy for, 191-192
Hyperpigmentation:
 Addison's disease, 44
 Cushing's syndrome, 39
 hemochromatosis, 44, 46, 146
Hyperpituitarism:
 acromegaly and, 114-117
 Cushing's disease and, 1-11
 prolactin-secreting adenoma and, 125,
  143-145
Hyperprolactinemia (see also Prolactinoma),
  122-124, 143
Hypertension, 86
 aldosterone and, 12-20
 Cushing's disease and, 8
 pheochromocytoma and, 29-34
Hyperthyroidism, 79-86, 97
 apathetic, 88-89
 causes, 90-91
 factitious, 60, 84, 90
 ophthalmopathy and, 82
 propranolol and, 83-84
 treatment:
  anti-thyroid drugs, 83-84
  surgery, 84
  radioactive iodine, 83
Hyperthyroxinemia, 54-61, 79-92
Hypocalcemia:
 causes, 180
 hypomagnesemia and, 180
 hypoparathyroidism and, 180, 184
 treatment, 181-182
 vitamin D deficiency, 180-181
Hypocalciuria:
 acromegaly and, 118
 familial hypercalcemic, 195
 osteomalacia, 205
Hypoglycemia, 168-176
 alcohol-induced, 174
 diagnosis, 170-171
 factitious, 173-174
 fasting, 170
 glucose tolerance and, 175
 insulin-induced, 170-171

insulin-induced tolerance test, 275-277
 postprandial, 175
 sulfonylureas and, 173
 therapy, 170-172
Hypogonadism:
 amenorrhea and, 124-126
 estrogen therapy, 162, 166
 hyperprolactinemia and, 143-144
 hypopituitarism and, 113
 impotence and, 143
 testosterone therapy, 144
 workup:
  females (diagram), 165
  males, 142-143
Hypokalemia:
 algorithm, 18
 hyperaldosteronism and, 12-20
 ketoacidosis and, 212
 rhabdomyolysis, 14
Hypomagnesemia, 91, 180
Hyponatremia:
 Addison's disease and, 42, 44
 ADH and, 266
 diabetic ketoacidosis, 212
Hypoparathyroidism, 180, 184
 Albright's osteodystropy and, 253-254
 causes, 184, 254
 treatment, 181-184
Hypophosphatemia:
 hyperparathyroidism and, 193
 osteomalacia and, 184
 vitamin D deficiency and, 180, 184
Hypopituitarism, 146
 causes, 108, 113
 hypogonadism and, 113
 tests for, 275-277
Hypothyroidism, 100-107
 diagnosis, 102
 tests for, 58-60
 TRH, 256
 TSH, 102, 256
 therapy, 103-104

Impotence, 139-148
Incidental adrenal mass, 21-28
Infarction, pituitary, 108-113

INDEX 283

Insulin:
C-peptide and, 173
hypoglycemia and, 171-172, 232, 234
therapy:
diabetic control and, 244-245
home monitoring, 231-233
ketoacidosis and, 211-212
"sliding" scale insulin, 249
Insulinoma:
diagnosis, 170-172
treatment, 172
Iodine:
-induced hyperthyroidism, 88-92
-induced hypothyroidism, 91
radioactive:
treatment, 83, 90, 97
uptake, 82, 88, 96
Islet cell tumors, 39, 172

Jod-Basedow phenomenon, 88-92

Kallman's syndrome, 145
Ketoacidosis, diabetic, 207-213
clinical features, 207, 210
diagnosis, 210
treatment, 211-212
17-Ketosteroids:
adrenal carcinoma, 27
hirsutism and, 156
Klinefelter's syndrome, 145

Libido, 142
Licorice, 15, 17
Lipoatrophy, diabetic, 248
Lipohypertrophy, diabetic, 251
Lung carcinoma, ectopic hormone
production, 39-40, 265-266
Luteinizing hormone (LH) (see also
Gonadotropins):
hypopituitarism and, 145
polycystic ovaries and, 152-153
releasing hormone (GnRH), 153

Magnesium (see hypomagnesemia)
Malabsorption, vitamin D and, 180
Medic-Alert, 113
Medroxyprogesterone, 164-166, 203
Menopause:
estrogen treatment, 203-204
osteoporosis and, 197-206
premature, 201

Metanephrines, 32
Methimazole, 83
Metyrapone:
Cushing's syndrome and, 40
pituitary-adrenal axis and, 270-271
MIBG scan, 34
Mineralocorticoids (see Aldosterone)
Modigliani syndrome, 55
Mononeuropathy, diabetic, 215
Multiple endocrine neoplasia (MEN):
type I, 34, 189, 194
type IIa, 34, 189, 194
type IIb or III, 75-78
Multiple myeloma, 189, 200
Myxedema (see Hypothyroidism), 104

Neck masses, (algorithm), 54
Necrobiosis lipoidica diabeticorum, 226,
Nelson's syndrome, 6
Nephrocalcinosis, 191
Nephrolithiasis, 191
Neurological disorders:
compression neuropathies:
acromegaly, 118
diabetic, 215, 228, 238-239
hypothyroidism, 102
Norepinephrine (see also
Catecholamines), 23, 29

Obesity:
diabetes mellitus and, 220
Onycholysis, 79, 263-264
Osmolality, 133-134
dehydration test, 133-134
Osteomalacia, 181, 205
Osteopenia, 197, 200
Osteoporosis, 197-206
causes, 201
clinical features, 203-204
estrogens and, 203
laboratory findings, 205
therapy, 202-206
Ovaries:
amenorrhea (algorithm), 165
androgen production, 155-156
gonadal dysgenesis, 166
polycystic ovary disease, 149-154

284 INDEX

Pancreatic tumors:
ACTH-producing, 39
insulinoma, 172
MEN I, 189, 194
Parathyroid hormone (PTH):
assay of, 194
deficiency, 184
estrogens and, 192, 203
hypercalcemia, 189-192
hypocalcemia, 184
magnesium and, 180
osteitis fibrosa and, 191
phosphorus and, 184, 193
resistance, 253-254
vitamin D and, 181-185
Pemberton's sign, 55
Pentagastrin, calcitonin, 75
Phenobarbital, osteomalacia, 139
Pheoxybenzamine, 33
Pheochromocytoma, 29-35
MEN and, 34, 75, 189, 194
workup for, 32-33
Pituitary:
apoplexy, 108-113
assessment of reserve, 112, 275-277
Cushing's disease, 1-11
infarction, 112
surgery, 7, 110, 117, 126
Plummer's disease, 90
Plummer's nails, 263-264
Polycystic ovaries, 149-154
Polydipsia, diagnosis, 132-133, 210, 220
Polyglandular endocrine failure, 45-46, 106, 146
Porter-Silber reaction, 271
Potassium:
Addison's disease and, 44
aldosterone and, 12-20
replacement therapy in ketoacidosis, 212
urine, 14, 18
Prognathism, 114, 116
Prolactin:
adenoma, pituitary, 125, 143-145
amenorrhea and, 122-128
galactorrhea and, 122
hypothyroidism and, 124
Prolactinoma:
diagnosis, 124-127, 143, 152
therapy, 126-127, 144
Propranolol:
for hyperthyroidism, 83-84

pheochromocytoma and, 33, 35
Propythiouracil (PTU), 83-84, 90
Pseudohypoparathyroidism, 253-254
Pseudopseudohypoparathyroidism, 254

Reactive hypoglycemia (see also hypoglycemia), 175
Reifenstein's syndrome, 167
Renin (PRA), 15-18
Resin uptake, T3, 58-60
Retinopathy, diabetic, 245-252

Sarcoidosis, 189-190
Schmidt's syndrome, 46
Sella turcica:
Hardy grades, 124
Sex hormone-binding globulin (SHBG), 157
Sheehan's syndrome, 166
SIADH (see also Antidiuretic hormone), 266
Sodium (see also Hyponatremia)
ADH and, 266
diabetic ketoacidosis and, 212
wasting, 44
Somatomedin, 116, 120
Somogyi phenomenon, 234
Spironolactone:
for hyperaldosteronism, 17
for hirsutism, 154
Stein-Leventhal syndrome (see Polycystic ovarian syndrome)
Stimulation tests:
ACTH (cosyntropin), 44, 156
dehydration, 133
L-dopa, 10
insulin-induced hypoglycemia (IIHT), 275-277
glucose tolerance test (GTT), 12, 220
metyrapone loading, 270-272
pentagastrin, 75
thyrotropin-releasing hormone (TRH), 256
Suppression tests:
dexamethasone, 4-6
glucose tolerance for GH, 117
Sulfonylureas:
for diabetes mellitus, 222-224
hypoglycemia and, 173-174

INDEX 285

Surgery:
  aldosteronoma and, 15-16
  adrenal adenoma/carcinoma and, 25, 27
  Cushing's disease and, 7
  diabetic patient and, 245-252
  gonadal dysgenesis, XY mosiacism, 166
  insulinoma and, 172
  hyperparathyroidism and, 191
  hypoparathyroidism and, 184
  parathyroid carcinoma, 193
  pheochromocytoma and, 33
  pituitary tumor and, 7, 117, 144
  thyroid and, 68-69, 76, 90, 97

Testes, size, 147
Testicular feminization, 159-163
Testosterone:
  deficiency, 143
  evaluation of impotence and, 143
  hirsutism and, 152
  plasma levels, 143
  producing tumors, 156
  production in women, 155
  replacement therapy, 155
Testosterone cypionate, 144
Testosterone enanthate, 144
Thiazides:
  diabetes insipidus and, 135
  hypercalcemia and, 189-190
Thymoma, ACTH-producing, 39
Throglobulin, 53, 69-70
Thyroglossal duct cyst, 52
Thyroid-binding globulin (TBG), 58-59
Thyroid biopsy
  fine needle aspiration, 65-66, 74
Thyroid gland:
  adenomas, 93-99
  carcinoma, 67-69, 75-76
  cysts, 52
  function in nonthyroidal illness (see
    Euthyroid sick)
  goiter:
    diffuse toxic, 79-85
    fat pad goiter, 48-56
    nontoxic, 52
    retroclavicular, 55
    simple, 52
    toxic multinodular, 86-92
  hemiagenesis, 98
  hyperthyroidism (see also
    Hyperthyroidism, 79-92, 97

hypofunction (see also hypothyroidism),
    100-107, 267-268
  nodules, 62-71, 73
  cysts, 52
    fine needle aspiration, 65-67, 70
    management of, 103-104
    radioactive iodine uptake, 82, 88, 96
    radionuclide scan, 65, 82
    tests (see also Thyroid hormones),
      58-61, 82
Thyroid hormones:
  antithyroid drugs, 83-84, 90
  contrast agents, radiographic, 88, 268
  decreased levels (see also
    Hypothyroidism), 102, 104-114
    267-268
  elevated (see also Hyperthyroidism),
    60, 79-92, 96
  euthyroid sick, 57, 267-268
  free thyroxine, 59-60
  replacement therapy, 103-104
  reverse T3 , 60, 268
  suppressive therapy, 68-69, 94
  thyroxine (T4), 58-59, 103
  triiodothyronine (T3), 60, 103
Thyroiditis:
  Hashimoto's, 52-53, 69, 105-106
  painless, 60, 85
Thyroid-stimulating hormone (TSH):
  hypothyroidism and, 102
  serum levels, 102, 104, 118, 256
  stimulation by TRH, 118, 256
Thyrotoxicosis (see Hyperthyroidism)
Thyrotoxocosis factitica, 84, 96
Thyrotropin (see Thyroid-
  stimulating hormone)
Thyroxine (see also Thyroid hormones)
  free, 59-60
  free thyroid index, 59-60
  replacement therapy, 103-104
  suppressive therapy, 68-69, 94
Transsphenoidal pituitary surgery, 7, 110,
    117, 126
TRH (see Thyrotropin-releasing hormone)
Triiodothyronine (see also Thyroid
  hormones):
  antithyroid drugs, 83-84, 90
  elevated serum levels, 97
  low serum levels, 268
  resin uptake, 58-59
  reverse, 60, 268

286 INDEX

Trousseau's sign, 180, 184
TSH (see Thyroid-stimulating hormone)
Turner's syndrome, 164, 166

Underbite, 114-121
Urine:
 aldosterone in, 15
 calcium in, 118, 195, 205
 catecholamines in, 25, 32
 cortisol in, 4-6, 44
 17-hydroxycorticoids, 4-10, 271
 17-ketosteroids, 27, 156
 metanephrines, 25, 32
 osmolality, 133
 potassium in, 14, 18
 vanillylmandelic acid (VMA), 25, 32
Uterus, absent, 164

Vagina, absent, 164
Vanillylmandelic acid (VMA), 25, 32
Vasopressin (antidiuretic hormone),
 129-138, 266
Virilization:
 adrenal hyperplasia, 4-6, 156
 adrenal tumors, 156
 ovarian tumors and, 155-156
 polycystic ovaries and, 152-154
Vitamin A intoxication, 189
Vitamin D:
 deficiency, 180
 intoxication, 182, 189
 malabsorption of, 180-181
Vitamin D2 (ergocalciferol), 182
VMA (vanillylmandelic acid), 25, 32

Water deprivation test, 132-134
Wolff-Chaikoff effect, 91

X-Linked hypophosphatemic vitamin D
 resistant rickets, 205